Energetics of Endo

A JOURNEY TO UNCOVER DEEPER MEANING BEHIND ENDOMETRIOSIS & INFERTILITY

AUBREE DEIMLER

Energetics of Endo
A journey to uncover deeper meaning
behind endometriosis & infertility
Copyright © 2019 by Aubree Deimler

All rights reserved.

The information presented herein is
not medical advice and is not intended to
diagnose, treat, cure or prevent any disease
and should not be used as a substitute for
the advice of a physician, therapist,
or other licensed health practitioner.
The content of this book is for general information only.
Please consult your doctor for matters
pertaining to your specific health and diet.

To contact the author please visit
peacewithendo.com

Cover art by: Dragan Bilic

ISBN: 978-0-578-21419-1

Dedication

To the Fantastical Kate Patchett. Thank you for lighting the way back to my soul purpose.

Contents

Forword

When I look at Aubree's energy, I see a stoic and masterful soul. If you venture for a moment into what I call "Spirit Space", you'll see a being who is unwavering and steadfast in her vision. In her hand, she holds a wand tipped with a small orb of multi-colored glass, which shines a light from within. Dragonflies hover around her as she stares out into the vastness of all that exists. With a steady hand, she weaves images into a tapestry depicting a deep inner journey filled with memories, soul desires, and spiritual exploration.

Write. Create. Be.

Aubree came home to her soul purpose through the act of writing this book.

It didn't happen overnight. Aubree was cracked wide open by the call to pay attention to what shaped her life, to allow the suffering she endured in her body to show her the way, to reach into her fears, and extract the truth of her soul. She discovered the interconnectedness of events, messages, and experiences, and their importance in bringing her to a place where she craved release from pains of the past — pains of a body betraying the soul. It took many steps, and much time for her to integrate each revelation. But with raw honesty, and incredible courage, she released the suffering.

It is through the lens of her personal story that you witness a woman discovering and unfolding the multi-dimensional nature of her soul experiences. The ultimate manifestation of disease in the soul is a physical pain. Aubree's quest to live with endometriosis, free of traumatic pain and suffering, led her to examine several layers of her being, from her inner child and parental connections, to the desire for a child of her own, and on to the imprints on her mind and body from sexual trauma, past life influences, and energy healing experiences.

This time of searching and learning ushered her into a space of vulnerable writing and the ability to create with clarity. Now, in the gorgeously tender *Energetics of Endo*, Aubree is openly sharing her story. She took matters into her own hands, finding her way through various techniques and healing modalities, the most impactful of which was expanding her psychic palette. I truly believe that through this book, Aubree will inspire women to dig for deeper understanding of their own innate, intuitive, healing power.

Kate Patchett
Visionary Soul Coach

Introduction

I struggled with excruciating pain during my periods from the start and was told over and over again that it was normal, that it was part of being a woman. Except I didn't notice my friends struggling like I did. My family doctor offered a high dose of Ibuprofen and sent me on my way, yet Ibuprofen didn't come close to touching the pain.

When I was 17, I got on birth control pills. That did help with the pain I had with my periods, but it came with other side effects. I started to experience digestive issues: bloating, constipation, gas, etc. I'd also started to question the impacts on my mental health. I never felt right when I took them. They gave me serious, crazy mood swings. I was easily upset, angered, and depressed. It was like once I reached a certain point, I snapped.

I got off the pill late in my twenties shortly before Ryan and I married. The pain with my periods returned with a vengeance along with a series of other symptoms like pain during and after sex, abnormal bleeding, cysts, and digestive distress.

"I wonder if you have endometriosis."

A co-worker was the first to mention the word to me after I'd missed another day of work when my period started.

"My friend has it and she gets really painful periods. Well, she pretty much has pain all the time."

Endometriosis (or endo for short) is a condition in which cells that are similar to those that line the uterus (the endometrium) become displaced and attach themselves to different organs. These out of place cells react like they're part of the uterus. So, with a normal menstrual cycle, they get thicker as the endometrium gets thicker. When menstruation happens, those displaced cells have nowhere to go. They aren't able to shed like they would if they were part of the womb. Instead, they inflame and hurt like hell. As those cells become increasingly agitated, your body tries to heal them with scar tissue. This can create painful adhesions that pull, twist, and stick between organs, causing further chronic pain.

After almost two decades of painful periods, how had I never heard of endometriosis? I'm grateful that my friend noticed and spoke up. Her words led me to Google, which led me to support groups, which led me back to the doctor's office. I had all the symptoms. Why hadn't endometriosis been mentioned all these years?

And what had that done to my subconscious? I expressed the pain, but it wasn't heard. It was shoved off as a normal part of being a woman. Subconsciously these messages taught me to distrust my senses and my developing body. It also brought self-esteem issues. My voice wasn't heard. This brought feelings of invalidation. My voice didn't matter. I stopped speaking up, until the pain made it so I was screaming. Something was wrong. I knew it. This was not normal.

I went to see my gynecologist to bring up this growing suspicion of endometriosis. After spending months researching on the Internet, and being a fly on the walls of support groups, it felt clear to me it was a real possibility. The wait to see her was long and the office was full of the pregnant bellies of women awaiting ultrasounds. I'd only just discovered endometriosis, and the reality that it could impact my body's ability to have a child. Sadness crept through me as my mind absorbed the possibility that I could never be one of those pregnant mothers.

By the time I got back to see the doctor I was extremely emotional. I was days from the start of my period, so I was already sensitive. At the end of the consult, when she confirmed that endometriosis was a possibility, I broke down in tears.

"Chronic pain is hard," she said.

Before I left, she presented me with a prescription for anti-depressants. I didn't mention feeling depressed. I was feeling overwhelmed with the notion of living with a chronic condition that could steal my chances of having a child of my own. After waiting for forty-five minutes, surrounded by pregnant bellies, it was understandable that I was upset. Yet those emotions were readily numbed with a prescription pad.

It's of no doubt the pain that comes with endometriosis is not only physical. There are emotional components that must be addressed and released. But it's easier said than done, especially when those feelings may have been pushed down or numbed for years. That was the case for me.

I learned early on how to numb both the physical and emotional pain. As a child, growing into a young woman, I went to the doctors when illness arose. I relied on the doctors to help get me better. I went to them, told them my symptoms, and took what was prescribed with little question. I'd pop the pills and move on. The problem, or symptom, would go away for a while, until it sprung up again. It was like trimming off leaves of a dying plant without addressing the roots, the soil.

Those trips to the doctor, and expectations of a prescription, conditioned me to continue seeking out something to numb the pain. I covered up negative feelings with different types of stimulates that made me feel better for a while. Most of the time that meant pills, alcohol, sugar, chocolate, or shopping. When the symptoms or emotions came back, I numbed them again. I was conditioned; feel pain ... get numb.

I think that decision was based on a subconscious fear. I didn't want to face the pain. I didn't want to feel bad. I just wanted it to go away — now.

My conditioned responses wore thin once the pain stopped going away. Even more so when the pills started to cause new symptoms, usually in my stomach. The toss up then became which type of suffering to tolerate.

Then it all came crashing down. A storm collided with a painful surgery that led to confirmation of endometriosis in my body: a chronic condition that I couldn't numb. It was too big, all-consuming.

The surgery provided visual evidence for all the pain I'd suffered through. There was a reason, it wasn't all in my head, it wasn't normal. I struggled for so long and had never heard of this condition. How was that possible?

I wasn't keen on the choices of treatment offered to me from the doctors: hormones, surgery, anti-depressants. No. I wasn't going to go that way. The answers I sought weren't available in the westernized medical system. I had to explore elsewhere. The decision to forge a new road to self-healing was carried by a strong belief that I could feel better with endometriosis.

I set out to find a holistic solution for this mysterious condition.

I was grateful for the connections I made online with other endo sisters who were following the same path. This helped me gather ideas. As I got into the world of alternative wellness and nutrition, however, I soon got confused.

There were so many things to try, so many suggestions. I updated my food and, since I'd been accustomed to taking a pill from the doctor, I shifted to buying cabinets full of supplements, powders, shakes, oils, and whatever. Soon I was overwhelmed and broke, caught up in a continued quest to stop the pain, to "fix" myself. I was impatient. I still just wanted to feel better, now. I was rushing, trying everything, and in turn, I wasn't sure what was working.

I'd missed a vital step to self-healing: awareness.

So, I stopped, stepped back, and asked myself the most important question on the journey to healing ... how do I *feel?* How often did I check in after I ate a meal, or *while* I ate the meal? When I woke up in the morning, when I introduced a new supplement ... *how do I feel?* After spending time around someone, being in different environments, when I didn't sleep enough ... *how do I feel?* When I ate too much sugar, or drank alcohol, or ate hot wings, or a home cooked meal and a super food drink ... *how do I feel?*

This check-in with myself helped build awareness and was pretty revolutionary for me. I wasn't used to asking myself how I felt. All I recognized was pain and that I wanted to make it stop. I didn't put the connection to the cause, because I wasn't connected to myself. When I tuned in, I discovered what choices impacted me, what made me feel good, and what triggered pain.

I started to listen to the messages of my body.

My exploration into managing endometriosis holistically turned into a passion and purpose to help other women with endo feel better, too. I received health coach training from the Institute for Integrative Nutrition (IIN), where I was trained on more than one hundred different dietary theories. My education equipped me with extensive knowledge in holistic nutrition, personalized coaching, and preventative health. Since graduating from IIN in 2014 with my health coaching certification, I've helped other women with endometriosis naturally manage pain, increase energy, and find peace with endo.

I share more about the steps I took on my healing journey and how you can follow suit in my first book, *From Pain to Peace with Endo*.

As a result of all the changes I'd made since my official diagnosis in 2011, I felt better most of the time. But there were still flare-ups and pain with my periods that rocked my world. That was frustrating to me. I felt like I was doing everything right, yet I'd hit a wall in my healing progress. The severe pain with my periods was a major disruption in my life. The experiences were traumatic and left behind feelings of fear and deep sadness.

Also, as I approached the mid-point of my thirties, I hadn't been able to hold onto a pregnancy. I watched the women in my life become mothers, and I waited, wondering if it would be my turn. The years of dealing with infertility had taken their toll. I felt misunderstood, and carried around bitterness that weighed down my heart space. I was tired of feeling that way.

I'd been pregnant a few times, but the new life didn't stay. Why? My intuition hinted that there were bigger blocks present. This was reflected back to me in conversations I had with other IIN health coaches over the years, as chakras and energy flow entered my vocabulary. These were new concepts to me. I hadn't considered the role of energy before.

I'd spent years addressing the physical part of my being with diet, exercise, supplements, etc., but I'd only touched the surface of my energetic "body", or the greater spiritual part of my Self.

Everything that's alive pulsates with energy. It surrounds you and carries emotional energy created by both your internal and external experiences, both positive and negative. Emotions are energy.

Every thought travels through your biological system, activating a physiological response. Some thoughts are more powerful than others. Experiences that carry emotional energy include your memories, beliefs, relationships, and traumatic experiences. The emotions from these experiences encode into your biological system.

Research from neurobiologist Dr. Candice Pert proved that the same kinds of cells that manufacture and receive emotional chemistry in your brain are also present throughout your body. Your emotions reside physically in your body, interacting with your cells and tissues. Your body contains a history of every event and relationship. This history contains your strengths, weaknesses, hopes, and fears.

The flow of energy inside, commonly described in the alternative health world as Chi, Spirit, Shakti, or Prana (life force) can get blocked up with pain, trauma, and fear. If too much of this energy builds up you feel depressed, tired, uninspired, and hopeless. When energy can't flow, there's darkness.

When you find a way to release the pain that's inside, you create space for energy to flow. Without blockages, energy flows freely. In order to break down these blockages, the pain must first be acknowledged, felt, and released. In short, you have to feel to heal.

It's easier said than done. Feelings weren't something I always wanted to deal with. I'd been conditioned to numb any discomfort, internalizing most things, rather than addressing them, and avoiding negative feelings as long as I could.

That is until my body screamed at me and shook my nervous system with incredible pain. Endometriosis forced me to *feel*. The pain reminded me that I was alive, and it made me question why. Why am I here in a body that holds great pain? Why the suffering? Was there a deeper meaning behind the pain with endometriosis and infertility? Was there a bigger block that needed to be released?

These questions brought me down a path of deeper Self-exploration that led to the writing of this book. With pen and paper in hand, I dug deeper into my subconscious and allowed the truth to flow through the words. In the process I pinpointed greater fears, insights, and revelations.

It wasn't until I addressed the spiritual aspects of my being that things shifted in a big way. I experienced powerful physical changes from energy work I received, which peaked my curiosity. I was intrigued about the energetic side of things, and its influence with endometriosis.

As I opened up to this deeper exploration, fueled by intention, things started to fall into place. I was guided down a path of greater healing that I wasn't expecting. I was led to teachers, healers, and inspirational women that changed my life.

I feel blessed to have captured that story along the way, and even more so because you've made space in your life to read it. I hope it encourages you to consider the role of the energetic and spiritual side of things in your own life, and that it expands your definition of healing encouraging you to become aware of, and dig deeper into, the emotional components of your life with endo.

I also hope that my story serves as a mirror to the fire inside of you, of a power beyond measure, and that it encourages you to pause and listen to that intuitive voice inside, to express your truth, and connect with your soul energy.

I thank you again for taking the time to read mine.

Much Love.

How to use this book

Before you get started, I'd like to note one thing. I'm an avid reader, always have been. I share many of the books that I've read along the way in the story to follow. You may think to yourself, wow, how does she have time to read that much?

My college liberal arts education came along with a lot of reading and it forced me to learn how to do so quickly. Now that I have freedom to read whatever I want, I continue to consume six to eight books a month. It's habit.

Plus, I'm a writer, obviously, and the more I read, the better I write.

Please don't feel like you have to read all the books I mention, and please don't let it overwhelm you. I know not everyone has the time or desire to read like I do (though I'm grateful that your reading time is being shared with me now).

I mention the books because they helped to shape my perception and experience. For those who do want to explore these resources further, check out the reading list at the end of the book.

The bulk of this book is my personal story and exploration of the deeper meaning behind endometriosis and infertility. I've shared it in this anecdotal format because I feel like stories are more relatable than a bunch of dry information spewed at you (which I'm perfectly capable of doing too!)

Through the act of mirroring you can start to discover your own triggers and meaning behind your personal experiences. I've shared intimate details of my life because I'm sure that there are others who can relate. I want you to know that you're not alone.

At the end of my narrative I've included some clear action steps you can take to get started on your own journey of exploration into the energetics of endo.

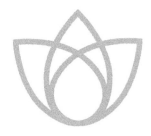

1. Freedom

*"But when we really delve into the reasons for why we
can't let something go, there are only two:
an attachment to the past or a fear of the future."*

~ Marie Kondo, The Life-Changing Magic of Tidying Up

*R*yan and I settled into a corner booth of the restaurant. I was happy to get away from the hustle and bustle of the morning breakfast crowd. I flashed him a smile, and even after a decade together, I still felt the swoon from the connection with his baby blue eyes.

The waitress arrived, and I was quick to order a pitcher of the hazelnut coffee. Ryan shook his head at me. I knew what he was thinking. I was running up the tab again with my caffeine addiction.

I settled back in the booth to review the menu. Out of the corner of my eye I spotted a stroller as it slid by the front of our table, stopping at the empty booth behind ours. I felt an ache at my heart when I saw the woman lift a tiny baby out and place it against her chest. A ripple of envy rolled through me.

My biological clock quivered. I was days away from my 34th birthday and still childless. The topic of fertility was to blame for much of the sadness that filtered my last December birthdays, mixed with the emotions of the holidays, and the quiet desire to grow our family as we watched everyone around us grow theirs. We were left behind, waiting and wondering if it would ever be our turn. Thirty-four. I'd reached the last year before the dreaded 35, the number that had implanted in my brain as the marking point of my declining fertility and transition to the "high-risk" category. Each year left behind meant fewer eggs, fewer chances.

After seven long years of trying, I wanted to believe I'd reached a pivotal point, directed towards acceptance. I may never bear a child. I tried to re-direct my thinking to a different, childless life. There were times when I was all right with that. I appreciated my freedom, sleep and sanity. Then little triggers came at random, unexpected times that reminded me of the grief held deep in my heart space.

Back in that restaurant, my eyes drawn to that woman with her newborn child, I felt all those emotions stir up again.

Ryan noticed my shift in energy. He glanced over his shoulder and looked back at me knowingly. I wasn't the only one with baby envy.

I tried to focus on my food, but the image was right in front of me. She was an off-duty employee at the restaurant and it appeared to be the first time she'd brought her beautiful newborn to work. All the other employees stopped by with squeals of congratulations.

Longest. Breakfast. Ever.

Once I escaped that suffocating situation and made it home to the quiet solitude of our upstairs bathroom, I released a flood of tears. My chest filled with pain. It was literal heartache.

While the past few birthdays had been spent in tears, 34 was different. There were no tears shed. I was too busy clearing space for new things. Maybe a baby, or perhaps another creation or imprint of my life that was moving forward, whether I wanted it to or not. Things weren't slowing down.

So, I spent my birthday discarding, clearing space for the new year of my life and whatever creations were to come. It started in my closet.

"Really? This is what you want to do on your birthday?" Ryan asked.

I smiled. Absolutely. It was the perfect time.

About a week prior I'd picked up a book called *The Life-Changing Magic of Tidying Up* by Marie Kondo. Marie's overall message is to create a home that's full of things that bring you joy. She suggested using the question as you go through the items in your home: *Does this bring me joy?* If the answer's no, then it needs to go. You deserve to be around things that bring joy in your life. Everything else is clutter blocking the way.

As I followed the exercises in the book, I had an eye-opening experience. I had too much stuff. I didn't realize how much until I saw it all piled together. It provided perspective and motivation for me to start discarding.

As I worked through mounds of clothes, I got better at picking up my guidance towards joy. It became immediate, instinctual. I get that may sound strange if you haven't tried it, but it really was this natural thing. The process helped build confidence and appreciation for the present moment.

Sometimes, you hold onto things because they are tied to something in the past, or are linked to fear of the future. What if I need it later? The bigger question: does it bring you joy *now?* If it's not serving you now and doesn't spark something in you, then get rid of it.

The entire process of discarding was freeing. It felt good to let go. I got rid of clothes that I'd carried around for years. I filled up seven extra-large garbage bags of stuff! Included were a tall stack of suits that no longer fit me. I'd lost a lot of weight when I changed my diet in an effort to naturally manage endometriosis. I'd struggled with the idea of getting rid of the suits for years, despite Ryan's persistence that they were no longer needed. What if I gained weight and needed to wear them again?

Fear. In reality, I didn't foresee a future of suits for me. More like yoga pants and leggings. If I needed a box of suits again in the future, I would deal with it then. I didn't need to hold onto something that might be. The decision-making process helped bring me back to the present. Does it serve me *now?*

Now. That's all there really is.

Truth be told, I didn't need the too-big clothes, but other women could surely find use for them, just like I had at one point.

While the whole process looked like spring-cleaning, it ended up being a profound start to 34. I initiated release from that which weighed me down. My jam-packed closet was causing silent stress. I'd transformed it into a space filled with clothes that I actually wanted to wear, that I felt good in, that brought me joy. It was a big purging in a little amount of time.

And it had only just begun.

A couple of weeks after clearing out my closets, Ryan and I rang in the New Year. I sat down on that first day and wrote out a long list of goals and resolutions. As I did so, I couldn't help but remember that I'd done the same thing the year before, yet many of the items failed to materialize.

I looked over the long list of new things I wanted to do in the new year and recognized my consistent overachieving pattern of thinking that I could do more than what was possible. There were only so many hours in the day, only so much energy I could extend. As a recovering Type A personality, that long list stressed me out and, in a way, set me up for failure, or severe fatigue. For years I'd believed that I could do more than I should. I'd pushed myself through and eventually burnt myself out. I was forced to stop and recover. That recovering included choices on where to spend my energy.

I crumpled up the long list of resolutions. This year was going to be different.

I remembered a talk I'd listened to by a beautiful soul named Danielle LaPorte. She taught the basics of writing out your Desire Map, which draws from one primary question: *how do I want to feel?* When you focus on answering this question, then you can carefully cultivate what to do with your time. You stop chasing goals and instead go after feelings. When you direct yourself towards how you want to feel, then it becomes easier to find focus.

How did I want to feel?

I wrote out a single word across the page — *freedom*.

I wanted to find freedom from the grief, sorrow, and anger that collected in my body after years of dealing with endometriosis and related infertility. I wanted to feel freedom from the pain that radiated from my lower back, up my spine, out to my hips, gathering at my neck and shoulders, making it ever harder to cope.

I wanted to find freedom from the thoughts that popped into my head that considered the role of death and how it might be a welcome escape from the pain — a simple slip down in the tub, so the water took over my breath, as pain collided with my abdomen, sending contractions and ripples of suffering. My uterus and its stray pieces wept. The pain was deep.

I wrote the word *freedom* big and bold and put it in a black picture frame next to my desk where I would see it every day, serving as a guidepost for how I wanted to feel moving forward.

I had little idea then of the magic that action would stimulate.

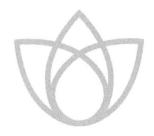

2. Awareness

"In the deepest sense, you free yourself by finding yourself.
You are not the one that periodically stresses out.
None of the disturbances have anything to do with you.
You are the one who notices these things.
Because your consciousness is separate and aware of these things,
you can free yourself."

~ Michael Singer, The Untethered Soul

A few weeks following my declaration for freedom, I woke up with horrible pain pulsing out of my abdomen. I ran my fingers along the inflamed area only to be met with bumps and ridges. What was that? It felt like a web stretched out inside. My mind swam with a loud thought — things are getting worse. Endometriosis, my nemesis.

I pulled myself up and trudged to the shower, hoping the warm water would help wash away the worry. It helped a little to ease my mind, but my body continued to tell its own story.

Ryan suggested we go out to lunch. It was a Saturday afternoon, so the restaurant was packed. We squished into the two-person table and my eyes fell down to the list of items on the menu. Frustration rose up. All the food was going to make me feel worse.

The pain flare filtered through my nervous system, rising tears in the corners of my eyes. I lowered my head, allowing my long brown hair to fall forward, shielding my face from what looked to be an emotional break.

Ryan noticed and asked the classic question that I didn't have a clear answer for.

"What's wrong?"

I sniffled in response, concentrating on the words on the menu, which were blurred from the onset of tears. It felt like everything was wrong. Life was wrong. My existence was wrong. I was exhausted. My body ached. Things were getting worse. These thoughts topped off with a cold hard fact: I was starving. As if on cue, the waiter appeared to take our order. I mumbled a half-hearted response.

"What's wrong?" Ryan repeated the question that lay unanswered.

"Nothing," I replied.

Classic response. It rang with disbelief as the tears broke the plane, sliding down my cheek to the top of the table.

Ryan let out an irritated sigh, "I don't know why we go out anymore."

He was obviously hungry, too.

The cut of his words added to all that was flowing through my body and mind and triggered me to jump from my seat. I couldn't stop the tears from pouring out. I sought refuge from the crowded space and bee lined it to the door. The cold air stung my face as I tore through the line of parked cars until I found ours.

I slipped into the front seat and shut the door behind me, sounding an echo in the secluded space. The stillness broke with my sobs. I cried out all the aggravation I felt in my body. The tears and convulsions from my stomach only added to the twists and turns of my insides. It felt like things were closing in, like I was wrapped up in a web of pain that wasn't going to go away. Fear was winning.

And I was hungry. My stomach growled in complaint, reminding me of the situation I left behind. I thought of Ryan sitting by himself with a plate across from him and an empty chair. I brushed away the tears, and took a look at myself in the visor mirror. The reflection was what I expected; my cheeks were pink and puffy. There was no way I would be able to hide that I was upset. I dreaded the thought of walking back inside.

Flipping back the visor, I sat back in the seat and closed my eyes. I took in the warmth of the sun through the windshield along with a couple of long deep breaths. This helped pull me back into my body and calmed things down. I remained in that space of calm for a couple of minutes before I jumped out of the car.

I kept my head low as I walked into the crowded restaurant.

I used my hair as a shield around my face, which wore an expression of the pain I worked so hard to hide. Some days it was harder than others.

I sat down across from Ryan, who was nearly done with his meal. I looked down at my abandoned plate of food, avoiding his eyes. The energy between us was tense. My stomach growled, urging me to eat what was in front of me. I put a bite of the cold food into my mouth and did my best to chew it down.

Ryan stopped the waiter as he walked by. "We're ready for the check," he said.

It seems I wasn't the only one who wanted to make a break from the restaurant. I struggled to eat a few more bites of food as Ryan paid.

"Did you want a box for that?" The waiter nodded towards my food.

I did my best to avoid eye contact, as I was aware of the message on my tear blotched face.

"No, thanks," I said, pushing the plate of cold food away.

The drive home hung heavy with silence. I directed my attention out the window at the passing landscape. The tears worked up again, sliding down like rain.

When we made it home, Ryan and I went our separate ways. He retreated to his man cave, and I made a break for the bathroom. It was there that most of my tears were shed. For whatever reason it felt safe to do it there, perhaps because it was a space where I wasn't disturbed. People respected the boundaries of a closed bathroom door.

I sat down on the top of the toilet, letting the tears stumble out again, wrecking pain and discontentment through my body. It felt like a large dam of emotions was breaking, emotions that needed to be felt. Those tears were full of pain and most of all ...

fear. I was afraid of what was going on in my body, afraid that things were getting worse, afraid that I'd never be able to have a child. I wasn't worth it. Those fears traveled through my nervous system, causing stress in an already stressful environment.

Eventually I broke from the confines of the bathroom in search of some type of solace, some way to calm down. On my escape outside to the back yard, I grabbed a book I'd just bought called *The Untethered Soul,* by Michael Singer.

I breathed in the crisp January air, and sat in one of the lawn chairs facing the sun, which was high in the sky. I flipped open the book and fell into the wisdom of Singer's words. They were just what I needed in that moment. He helped me witness the situation of pain from a new light, from a space of awareness.

The thoughts in my head, the voices of my mind, those weren't really me. My mind was what was causing problems, gathering fear. The feelings coursing through my body were part of my human existence and experience, but they weren't the real "me".

In that moment I was reminded that there's a greater part of myself that's not of the physical. This higher Self, or soul part of my being, is directed connected to God, the Divine, Source, the Universe ... however you describe it. It was the one who listened to these thoughts. This higher part of my Self saw me, and most importantly, it understood.

Singer's words, and my meditative time out in the sun, helped me to see that the pain needed to be acknowledged. I'd been pushing it down, until the volcano erupted.

In the warmth of the sun, the pain was recognized. I came back to my breath in the here and now, tuning into my feelings in that moment. I felt things as they were, which allowed those feelings to move through, rather than gather inside of me. I recognized that the thoughts in my head were only making things worse. I took a moment to relish in the space between them. Silence and sunshine helped calm my nerves.

In the days to follow, I continued to pull in small bits of *The Untethered Soul,* and each time I took in Singer's words, I felt something stir inside. His wisdom was exactly what I needed during that time and I think it no accident that I fell upon his book when I did.

Life was surrounding me with situations for growth, but it was up to me how to deal with it. I could permit the pain deep into my heart space, or I could allow it to pass through. I could live in fear of what could be, of that which I could not see, or I could accept the pain as part of this human existence, and release the fear of feeling all of it.

No more running.

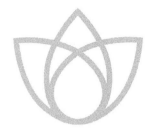

3. Sensitivity

"The goal here is to tune into ourselves better. The better we know ourselves the easier it is to distinguish what's ours and what's not. As sensitives, this is a challenge given how deeply we connect to others, especially loved ones."

~ Gigi Miner, The Highly Sensitive Empath:
Feeling Skinless in a Sandpaper World

*I*t was a gray February day. Clouds kept the light from shining through, in alignment with the news to come. I heard Ryan on the phone in his man cave and could tell from his side of the conversation that something was wrong. I could feel the energy shift even though I was on the floor above him. My heart picked up in my chest. I felt anxious, the kind of anxious that made me want to start pacing the room, which was probably exactly what he was doing.

The conversation continued for a while before Ryan hung up. Silence ensued. I waited in it. My curiosity encouraged me to get up and see what was wrong, but I stayed put. I knew he would come when he was ready to share.

As soon as he walked into the room, his face confirmed what I'd already suspected. Something was definitely wrong.

Ryan's voice was shaky. One of his good friends had committed suicide the night before. He was someone Ryan had developed a strong relationship with, playing Xbox together online, and having conversations late into the night.

The experience of loss by suicide ran deep in Ryan's history, and the passing of his friend brought up old scars that opened up and bled out. Needless to say, this caused a disturbance of energy in our home. I picked up on the sadness, even though I hadn't personally known his friend.

It forced me to reflect a lot on where the decision to commit suicide comes from. It must be from a desperate desire to put a stop to pain one fears will never end, that split-second moment when a person feels like there's no other way out. Emotional pain could be worse than the physical. The energy of darkness can be intense. I knew it well.

But even with suicide, the pain doesn't end. Instead it's

multiplied and spread out to all those who lost, to all those who will forever wonder: *Why?*

Pain. Guilt. Abandonment. It conjured up a lot.

"Let's go get some food," Ryan suggested.

I didn't feel like food. I felt sick, but I could tell that his suggestion had a deeper message — he needed to get out of the house. He needed some air.

We sat at the back of the sushi restaurant that had floor to ceiling windows, giving us a grand view of the gray day. I listened to him try to make sense of the situation. He worked through the common questions: when, where, and how. Yet one question remained unanswered. It was the question that is never answered with suicide: *Why?*

"I thought I was getting through to him," he said.

Ryan recounted long conversations they'd had about life, love, and loss. I remembered some of them well, or at least, the half of the conversations that I heard as Ryan spoke into his Xbox headset. He was always drawn toward helping others that were struggling because he'd felt so much pain and loss in his own life.

"You should write a song about it," I suggested. I could tell that he needed a way to release the pain that was radiating toward me. I felt sick.

Later that afternoon, I heard his guitar coming through the floor. I nodded in silent recognition of him taking my suggestion. As the night wore on, that guitar pieced into an organized rhythmic compilation. He wrote out words that reflected the pain, a part of his soul. It was a piece of art, an expression of the hurt, and absolutely beautiful. He titled it, *'When Angels Cry'.*

"I'm going to give it to his family to play at the funeral," he told me.

I nodded silently.

"I need to get it perfect before then," he said.

Over the course of the next couple days, I listened to that perfection play out, over and over again. There was a point when I had to block my ears, not because of the song itself, but because of the big influx of emotion that flared through me.

My entire body ached. Tears flowed out. This happened simultaneously as Ryan bled out his grief in that composition, fueled by the tremendous loss of a friend, and past emotions that came up from the loss of his father, who had also taken his own life.

"Writing the song was helpful," he said, but the process had come with a lot of intense emotions. He cried, burrowed, and dug deep into all that was stirred up by this loss.

I couldn't help pulling in the sadness that vibrated from the sounds and emotions Ryan transferred into his music. My body picked up on that energy in a big way. I physically felt the pain from his experience, and I'd recently learned why. I'm a highly sensitive empath (HSE), I pick up on other's energy. Once I became aware of this, I started to understand better why I am the way I am.

There are two parts to the HSE equation: highly sensitive plus empath. You can be a highly sensitive person without being an empath, while all empaths are highly sensitive.

As a highly sensitive person, I have a hair-trigger nervous system, and am aware of subtleties in my environment. I'm sensitive to noises, smells, colors, and other stimuli. All of this can lead to anxiety, especially in social situations. I'm easily overwhelmed, have a hard time watching scary or violent movies, and am easily moved by emotional scenes.

An empath is one who's capable of feeling the emotions or physical symptoms of others, even if you're not going through the same situations or events (This is not to be confused with basic empathy. All of us have the ability to empathize with another). An empath can literally feel the anxiety, sadness, and emotional pain from another, as if they were directly experiencing the same. This makes it difficult to assess how you feel, and it makes it harder to be around others that are in pain.

I experience aches and pains from my loved ones, or other people that are around me. I pick up on certain energies and emotions, and may have a hard time concentrating when others are around, or I feel overwhelmed easily while hanging out with others, especially in crowded places.

The challenge is in separating myself from other people's emotions long enough to recognize my own. When I'm on my own, I feel a sense of calm and normalcy. It's vital for me to have space to re-group alone, to tune into my own energy so I can distinguish it from others. It also means that I must express myself creatively or I start to get really cranky.

As Ryan released the sad suicide song on his guitar, I went for my notepad. I had to find solitude, to sort out the emotions that were coursing through me. I needed to draw my own boundaries.

I escaped into the backyard and used my breath to help pull me back into my own body, into the present moment. The cold February air helped with that. I wrote out how I was feeling, to help sort out if the sadness was mine or not. My heart was aching.

This topic of being highly sensitive has come up before in endometriosis support groups that I've been part of, which got me wondering if being an HSE is common with endo. It would make sense if so. The womb is a powerful space. It's the place of new life. It's the place that births our creative feminine energy, our intuition. What happens when cells that resemble the inside of this powerful organ end up all over your body? It's no wonder we're so sensitive.

Endometriosis impacts your nervous system in a pretty drastic way, putting your body on full alert. Your nervous system is what picks up on outside energy, connecting you to it. There's a delicate interplay with your nervous system and your endocrine system. Your nervous system controls balance through nerve impulses, while your endocrine system releases hormone messengers into your blood stream. This becomes worse if you face a life tragedy, like the death of a loved one.

Many women I've met with endo have experienced high stress situations at an early age, which altered the functioning of their nervous system later. Some of us were born more sensitive to stress. This sensitivity starts as early as the environment you experienced when you were in the womb, followed by childhood. If you grew up in an environment with lots of anxiety, fighting, or stressful events, then your body was impacted. The result? You're more sensitive to stress and likely more sensitive to the stress of others.

I had to learn to be selective with my energy. I'm easily drained when I'm around negative energy, from either people or events. For this reason, I very rarely read the mainstream news. I need space alone to refuel and restore, especially after a big social gathering, more so if it was something sad, like a funeral — or days of hearing a sad suicide song.

On the opposite spectrum, I also pull in positive energy and inspiration from others. That's the energy I want to be around. Once I became more aware of this, I could sense my intuition about situations almost immediately. Intuition is a powerful thing, especially on the journey to self-healing.

Empaths *feel* the world around them, which lends us to being innate healers, including the ability to heal ourselves. We are drawn to professions where we can help others. I think that's natural. If you pick up on the energy of others, it makes sense to want to help heal other's pain. That way we get to feel better, too. It has been my natural inclination to want to remove the pain from others around me, and as a result I often took it up on myself, as a channel of sorts, which easily led to exhaustion.

Turns out that my new path of feeling everything that came up was harder than expected, especially when those feelings weren't mine. What else had I picked up along the way?

4. Family

"Recent developments in the fields of cellular biology, neurobiology, epigenetics and developmental psychology underscore the importance of exploring at least three generations of family history in order to understand the mechanism behind patterns of trauma and suffering that repeat."

~ Mark Wolynn, It Didn't Start with You

The phone rang three times before he picked up.

"Happy birthday, Dad," I said.

"Thanks Aubree."

After exchanging a bit of small talk our conversation shifted to the discussion of books. As an avid reader I had three to four books going at a time: self-help, spiritual, wellness, business, fiction, etc. My attention span was short, so I filled my mind with a bunch of different things that moved me forward on my intentional path to *freedom*.

"Now Discover Your Strengths," I told him, as I eyed a self-help book that was acting as a support for papers and notebooks amid the chaos of my desktop.

"It's based on the findings from the Gallup StrengthsFinder assessment. Through a series of questions, it pinpoints your natural strengths. I took the test about ten years ago at my job, and re-took it this week. My strengths came back almost identical ... except for one," I said.

"What was different this time?"

I reached for the book and flipped to the pages I'd dog-eared.

"I was competitive. Now I'm strategic."

My father chuckled, "That competitive streak runs in the family. What are some of your other strengths?"

"Learner, Intellection, Analytical, and Achiever."

"You get the achiever part from me," he said.

I nodded. He was right. My father had always worked hard. At an early age he joined the Air Force and was conditioned by discipline, order, and routine. As a child, I watched that play out into his daily routines, which included many household tasks like cooking and cleaning. There was always order to things.

Shortly after I graduated from high school, my father took on a life of leadership and service in the Catholic Church. This role took a lot of his time, especially on the weekends, so it became harder to connect. He was around less, and when he was present, his energy was often low. At the time, it felt like he was slowly slipping away.

"I've read that the over achiever type can come from a desire to be seen and accepted. It can stem from childhood," I said. My heart picked up in my chest, as my words hung vulnerable in the air. What daughter doesn't want to be seen and accepted by her father? I certainly did.

"That drive to always be doing something comes from an underlying fear of losing control," I continued.

"That makes sense," he replied.

"I have issues delegating tasks," I continued, "because I have issues giving over the control. I want it to be done right."

"I know what you mean," my father agreed. "I have issues delegating tasks too. I figure that it's easier to do everything myself."

"Because then you'd have to give up control," I probed.

"You're right," he said.

I smiled. It felt good to have a conversation with my dad that stepped outside everyday small talk. Our conversations were usually straight to the point, cut off. It felt good to have his attention for a while.

"This can be worse when you experience trauma as a child," I told him.

"That makes sense, too. My mother died when I was six," my dad said.

Six. It was the same age Ryan was when his father died. I'd been witness to the impacts of that loss that weighed heavily on Ryan's world, playing out in a similar 'achiever' personality. In that moment I understood what it meant when they say women tend to marry men like their fathers.

"I bet that was hard."

I could sense the energy shift on the other side of the phone. I put a hand over my heart.

"Have you thought about writing about it?" I suggested the same advice I gave to Ryan, and to anyone dealing with a lot of emotions about something; find a way to express it.

My father's an amazing writer. The magic of his words spilled into letters and handwritten notes to me over the years. He had a way with words.

"I have an outline for a book."

I smiled.

"I hope you write it," I said.

After we hung up, my father's sadness lingered with me. I thought more of this woman, my grandmother, whom I'd never met, and something told me I needed to know more.

Shortly after that conversation with my father, I came across an article that included an excerpt from a book by Mark Wolynn titled, *It Didn't Start With You: How Inherited Family Trauma Shapes Who We Are.* I believe it was placed in my path with divine timing. It explained how emerging trends in psychotherapy point beyond the traumas of the individual to include traumatic events in the family and social history, as part of the whole picture. The article intrigued me enough to immediately order the book.

The book explored the influence of past family trauma on your genetics and subconscious mind. These tragedies included things like abandonment, suicide, war, and the early death of a child, parent, or sibling. These traumatic events can send shock waves of distress that cascades from one generation to the next. Wolynn provides compelling examples of people who experienced similar trauma as their ancestors, generations later. The trauma repeated until it was identified and dealt with.

To help identify this underlying trauma, Wolynn's a strong proponent for examining the language and words you use. He provided different writing exercises in the book. I picked out some words that could shine a light on potential past trauma. One that was duplicated in my writing was "express". This caught my attention.

Both of my parents are extremely introverted. Growing up there was little verbal expression, especially when it came to deeper emotions. My parents rarely fought in outward expression, instead they tended to retreat. Silence followed for inner reflection. This conditioning carried forward in my own relationships later in life. I had a hard time expressing what I needed. I got mad about things I felt like others should just know, even though I didn't say what I was thinking. I repeated the learned behavior. I got angry, and then withdrew.

Growing up, I didn't learn how to express my emotions. I was conditioned to bury and internalize them. I locked things up, didn't talk about how I felt. I didn't really know how to until I met Ryan. He opened up and encouraged me to speak my truth.

Further writing exercises in *It Didn't Start with You* lead me to discover my greatest fear — *I'll lose control.*

I thought back to the conversation with my father and the sadness I detected from the loss of his mother, and the loss of control that was stimulated by that experience. Was that a key part of this underlying fear of my own? Was it passed down to me?

I'd struggled thus far in my life with physical pain from endometriosis, a condition labeled incurable, one that will spread, one that threatens my fertility, one that felt so out of control. This fear was underlying.

I'll lose control.

All of this stirred up a strong realization that I didn't know my roots very well. Why am I the way I am? Why do I hold these fears? Growing up I had slim to no communication with my family, outside of my parents, brothers, and maternal grandmother. I didn't really know where I came from. Was there more to it? My curiosity prompted me to set up a conversation with my parents.

We sat around the kitchen table in their home, my father on one side, my mother on the other, and me in between. I'd lent little explanation for why I'd set up the meeting, only vaguely saying, "We need to talk." I explained how I was writing this book in explorations of internal blocks that were keeping me from getting pregnant. I explained my voyage of self-discovery, as best as I could up until this point. I relayed the information I learned from *It Didn't Start with You* on how past trauma can carry forward into future generations, and pointed out two obvious traumas that came from both sides of my immediate lineage.

I could sense the sadness as my father spoke about his mother and this revolving wonder of how his life would have turned out if she hadn't died. I cried along with him, big fat tears streaming down my cheeks. In that moment I felt the great heaviness of this loss. I'm not sure that the loss of a parent ever goes away.

For me, it was the loss of a grandmother. How would my life have been different if she was around? Shortly after she died my grandfather re-married, and had several more children with, a woman who was much younger. My dad didn't get along well with his stepmother. He recounted stories that relayed feelings of blame, isolation, and resentment.

I didn't know my father's family. I didn't know my grandfather outside of a card I got every year for Christmas with some cash. I didn't know my aunts or uncles. There was a great disconnection and with that, I sensed that there was a great amount of grief. How much of that pain was passed down to me?

My father's story of loss and what followed in his young life sounded very similar to the experiences of the man I spent my life with, Ryan, who connected me on a greater spiritual level. I could see similarities between my father and husband's story.

In his book, *It Didn't Start with You*, Wolynn explained how you often unconsciously choose a partner who will trigger your inner wounds so that they too can see, own and heal themselves. Relationships serve as a perfect mirror to what's unfinished at the root of the other.

After wiping away tears, I turned my attention to the other side of the table, where grief was also present. My mother lost her father when she was young. He was another missing part of the picture. Who was this man?

"What do you remember about your dad?" I asked.

"He was in the military during WWII," she said, "When he got back from the war, he never talked about it. We weren't allowed to talk about it either."

War was a definite traumatic experience. I could only imagine what my grandfather saw during that time when millions of people died because of what they looked like or what they believed in. Did he have a way to release all the turmoil that came from his time overseas? My grandfather died shortly after he came home from the war. He had stomach issues. Maybe he couldn't stomach what he'd seen — he didn't know how to digest it all.

"I was 12 when he died," she said.

The number 12 caught my attention. That was my age at the time of my first period, when the pain in my life really started, horrible pain at the center of me. 12 years old was an awkward time of transition to womanhood. I couldn't imagine dealing with all that on top of the enormity of losing a parent.

"How did you feel after he died?" I asked.

My mother deflected her own sadness, instead bringing up a memory of my grandmother broken-hearted at the funeral. I could only imagine the grief.

When my grandmother was still alive, she often spoke of the great love she had for my grandfather and how his death shook up her world. When she got close to her own death, aging into a life with dementia, losing her short-term memory, I got glimpses into the long-term memories that stuck. Love and loss.

"Our relationship changed after my dad died. It brought us closer," my mother said. A pause followed, a silent memory of losing my grandmother only a couple of years prior.

"She was a strong woman," my mother said. "She was a single mom and went to college to become a teacher."

I think that my mother had to be strong too, not only because she lost her father, but also because she had to watch out for her mother. Perhaps she remembered this image of my grandmother at my grandfather's funeral because it was a reflection of her own grief. As she transitioned into being a woman, she looked up to her mother. She decided to be strong, just like her father did when he came home from war. What happens to a young girl when she loses her father's love at an early age, during a time when hormones change, and boys come into the picture? Her father's love was missing.

As I sat in between my mother and father, hearing for the first time the history of their losses, my body ached with lingering sadness. I think the trauma from both of my parents was a wound that carried forward into my subconscious. I felt the deeper trauma in my family's history that had been shoved down and numbed. I'm not sure it was fully processed before it was passed onto me. It was up to me to finally feel the pain, which needed to be felt in order to be released. That was the only way I was going to be free of it. My father described it as "empty space", a phrase that would be played out over again in my own life as I lived with my own "empty spaces."

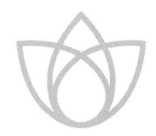

5. Chakras

"The chakras are vertically aligned, running from the base of the spine to the crown of the head, suggesting that we ascend toward the Divine by gradually mastering the seductive pull of the physical world."

~ Caroline Myss, Anatomy of the Spirit

$\mathcal{A}$s the year progressed and the weather outside grew warmer, I uncovered many lessons towards my intention for *freedom*. I knew more about who I was and where I came from. More importantly, I became more aware and in tune with the true "me", my higher Self. I felt connected to a higher spiritual vibe.

People fell into my path in synchronicity with information that took me closer to my desired feelings of *freedom*, and I continued to pay attention to those messages. One beautiful soul that came into my life was a woman named Steena Marie. I logged into Facebook one day, and was met with her live stream video. She immediately pulled me in.

Steena spoke of energy centers in the body called chakras. The word chakra comes from the Sanskrit word for wheel or vortex: a symbol of energy. Eastern philosophy teaches that there are seven different chakras arranged along the spinal cord. Energy flows along this pathway much like blood in the circulatory system.

These chakra energy centers are a driving force behind your physical existence. It bridges your worldly self with a higher consciousness and purpose in this earthly realm.

Blockages or energetic dysfunctions in these centers are believed to give rise to disorders. In order to help illness and disease this underlying energy source needs to be understood and balanced.

The chakra centers connect on a physical basis with your endocrine and nervous systems, and relate to a unique aspect of your mental, emotional, and spiritual well-being. Furthermore, each one is associated with a different color and earthly element.

1. ROOT

The first chakra is located at the base of your spine. Much like a tree's roots act as a base to stabilize it in the earth, the root chakra acts as a base for your body's energetic vibration. It's the root of you. The color of the root chakra is red, and its element is, predictably, earth.

Connecting with your adrenal glands and the coccygeal nerve plexus, the root chakra also governs your legs, feet, lower back, tailbone, and reproductive system. Psychologically, the root chakra deals with physical identity, stability, ambition, and self-sufficiency. It's based on innate energy concerning survival. It's what grounds you to this earth. This root energy connects to deeper ancestral energy and what psychologist Carl Jung referred to as the collective unconsciousness.

Issues with your root chakra can materialize as fatigue, poor sleep, lower back and sciatica pain, constipation, depression, and immune related disorders. Psychological and emotional issues can show as anger, fear, low self-esteem, and feelings of alienation.

When your root chakra is balanced you feel grounded, centered, independent, energetic, and strong.

2. SACRAL

The second, or sacral, chakra is located between your naval and pubic bone. Its associated color is orange, with water being its representational element.

The sacral chakra connects with your ovaries, splenic, and sacral nerve plexus, encompassing your reproductive organs, pelvis, large intestine, lower vertebrae, appendix, and bladder (all areas often burdened by endometriosis).

Psychologically, this energy center deals with a balance of mind and body, center of self, letting go, and going with the flow. It governs creativity, sensuality, sexuality, happiness, and joy. Emotional identity, desire, and personal relationship issues including expressing your needs and desires and the intimate act of giving and receiving, are all related to this second chakra.

Negative emotions block your sacral space. Physical issues in the chakra include fertility and other reproductive organ problems, menstruation difficulties, and problems with the kidneys and bladder. Mental issues related to a blocked sacral chakra include anxiety, stress, depression, self-punishing thoughts, and addiction.

When your chakra is balanced you feel creative, sensual, confident, and in flow with the energy of joy.

3. Solar Plexus

The third, or solar plexus, chakra is located above your navel, just below your rib cage. The color of the solar plexus is yellow, and its earthly element is fire, representing light and heat.

Your solar plexus connects with your pancreas and celiac nerve plexus, and reins over your digestive system, metabolism, liver, and gallbladder. Physical issues with your third chakra show up as diabetes, pancreatic and adrenal imbalances, arthritis, intestinal issues, anorexia, bulimia, and low blood pressure.

Psychologically, this energy center has to do with the establishment of healthy boundaries. It supports will power, self-assertion, transformation, and personal freedom. It's your connection with your sense of personal power and understanding of your higher Self.

Emotional blockages in your solar plexus manifest as a lack of self-esteem, timidity, depression, self-image issues, fear of rejection, inability to make decisions, judgmentalism, perfectionism, anger, rage, and hostility.

When your third chakra is balanced you feel energetic, confident, intelligent, decisive, and productive, with good digestion, and mental focus.

4. HEART

The fourth, or heart, chakra, is located mid-chest near your heart and lungs. The color of the heart chakra is green or pink, and the associated earth element is air, also represented as wind and gaseous matter.

Connecting to your thymus gland and cardiac nerve plexus, your heart chakra reigns over your circulatory and respiratory systems, along with your lymphatic and immune systems. Physical issues with your fourth chakra manifest as disruptions with your thoracic spine, upper back and shoulders, heart conditions, and asthma.

Psychologically, this chakra has to do with letting go, forgiveness, and emotional intimacy. Your heart space holds soul energy of hope, love, and peace, governs feelings of pure unconditional love, compassion, gratitude, self-acceptance, and equanimity. It also deals with social identity, forgiveness, wisdom, and deeper soul issues.

Emotional issues in this energy center show up as difficulty with love, lack of hope, compassion, and confidence, despair, moodiness, envy, fear, jealously, anger, and anxiety.

When your fourth chakra is balanced, you feel complete and whole, compassionate, friendly, optimistic, motivated, and outgoing.

5. THROAT

The fifth chakra is your throat chakra, which includes your entire neck region and your voice. Its color is blue, and its related element is ether, or the sky, space, and heavens.

Your throat chakra connects your thyroid and pharyngeal nerve plexus. It governs your throat, neck, ears, sinuses, respiratory system, and your voice. It has to do with sound.

Psychologically and emotionally, this chakra relates to deep communication, trust, and speaking your truth. It's connected with your sacral chakra in that it stimulates artistic development and creativity.

Your throat chakra encompasses taking responsibility for your needs, confession, faith, self-knowing and expression. When you have issues with this energy center, they come in the form of emotional dysfunction with faith, decision-making, personal expression, creativity, criticism, and addiction.

When it's balanced, you feel creative and centered, with positive self-expression.

6. THIRD EYE

The sixth chakra is your third eye, located between your eyebrows. Its color is indigo, and its element is your mind.

The sixth chakra connects your pituitary gland and carotid nerve plexus. It governs your endocrine and autonomic systems. Relating to your thoughts, intellect, opinions, and views, this energy center has to do with clear vision, intuition, and higher consciousness. Your third eye relates to your perception of self and awareness through meditation. It deals with self-knowledge, wisdom, insight, understanding, intuitive reasoning, and visualization.

Blockages manifest emotionally as judgment, evaluation, conception of reality, confusion, fear of the truth, and discipline.

When it's balanced, you feel intuitive and focused to a point where you can think reality into existence.

7. CROWN

The seventh and final chakra is your crown, located at the top of your head. Its associated color is magenta, and its element surpasses space and time.

Your crown chakra connects your pineal gland and meridian and cerebral cortex. It governs your central nervous system and upper spine.

This energy center relates to inspiration and connection to God, Source, the Divine, the universe, however you describe it. It's where you can find enlightenment, spiritual awareness, and intuitive guidance. Your crown chakra resonates as thoughts and has to do with space and unity.

Blockages in your crown space materialize as exhaustion and chronic sensitivity to light and sound. Emotionally, blockages show up as a lack of purpose, loss of identity, disbelief in spiritual realities, absence of trust, inspiration, values, and ethics, and sense of fear.

When your crown chakra is balanced, you feel one with the universe, open-minded, thoughtful, and intelligent.

After Steena did a review of the chakras on her live stream, she offered to do oracle card readings for whoever was watching. The cards were meant to serve as guidance. I expressed my interest in the comments and watched as she pulled two cards for me from a beautiful deck that she created herself.

One of the cards she pulled for me showed a simple message, "BE YOU." I listened as she described an energetic block in my root chakra and pelvic bowl area, and how past relationships were in need of healing. These blocks were heavy and were keeping me from moving forward.

As with many of the messages I'd received during the year, I took Steena's words to heart, and I believed her intuitive gift to be true. I was intrigued enough to schedule a one-on-one private reading with her.

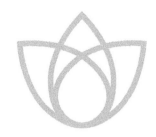

6. Pelvic Energy

"When a wound is witnessed its energy begins to change.
Instead of remaining held in the energy field of the body,
it becomes observable and moveable.
You can interact with it, dissipating its power or held energy.
Energy previously spent to contain the wound
is now available for use in another more conscious way."

~ Tami Lynn Kent, Wild Feminine

*B*efore our call, Steena tuned into my energy and sent over a drawing of how she saw my aura, the colored energy field that encircles your body. She was able to see the size, color, and type of this vibration around me, while tuning into my chakras and helping me balance what was off. Her analysis was spot on.

She told me that my root chakra looked wired like it was all over the place. That pretty much summed up how I felt at the time — flighty and unfocused. I bounced between tasks, often forgetting what I was doing halfway through. When your root is off, this impacts all the other chakras. If you don't have a steady base, everything else gets misaligned, too.

Steena also picked up on issues in my sacral region. She explained the dual nature of masculine and feminine energy in the body, and how imbalance of those energies often manifests in the sacral chakra. Symbolically and energetically, male energy is all about giving, while female energy is about receiving. This dichotomy is reflected physically in the pelvic space.

Masculine energy correlates to the right side of the body, and is more ordered, systematic, and driven. Feminine energy correlates to the left side of the body, and is more flowing, intuitive, and creative.

I had issues with the right side of my body. That was where most of my physical suffering was centered — a pocket of pain in my hip and lower back.

"Your solar plexus energy is pulling to the right," Steena confirmed, "That indicates an imbalance of male energy."

I knew she was right. I'd been doing too much, pushing myself too hard, dominated by the force of male energy which seeks always to get things done, and in turn I was depriving myself of much needed rest. I was giving, giving, giving to others but not leaving space for receiving. This was a common theme in my life. I was always doing something, because if I stopped, it felt like failure.

"Nurture yourself for at least ten to thirty minutes a day, twice a week. Show yourself that you can be trusted and follow through," she instructed.

"I can do that," I promised.

"Rotate your hips, sing, dance, express yourself," she suggested, "Yoga would benefit you greatly by grounding your energy and creating space to receive."

"Ok," I said, making a mental note to add that to my long list of things to do.

To help me find further balance in my sacral space, and within this dual nature of male and feminine energies, she recommended a couple of books: *Wild Feminine* and *Women Who Run With the Wolves*. I made note to add the books to my to-read list.

Steena explained the connection between the sacral, heart, and throat chakras, and how they were all related to expression and creativity. When she got to my heart chakra, she told me she saw it stretched way out, like my arms were open in a big hug.

"I'm a writer," I confessed.

"I could sense that about you," she said. "Your hands are direct extensions of your heart energy, but the way your heart energy is stretched, it's like you're spreading too much love, without returning enough for yourself."

Moving up to my throat chakra, she found a misbalance in my ability to communicate. Even though I was expressing myself through writing, I had issues with vocalizing, I struggled to stand up and speak up. My voice was another tool, a way to speak my truth, to give words to who I really was. I'd been so afraid to use it, silenced by insecurities.

Steena suggested tapping into my heart energy and allowing it to envelope me before speaking.

"Have voice affirming intuition. Speak your inner knowing. Do it in front of a mirror," she advised. "Offer loving words to yourself."

I tried the technique later that evening. Looking deep into my eyes within the reflection in the mirror, I searched for my truth. There's power in eye contact, especially when it's with yourself. It was like I was peering right into my soul.

"I love you," I whispered.

The main message I took away from my call with Steena was the need to stimulate the feminine energy of receiving. I needed to give attention to my inner, nurturing role, because I wasn't taking enough time for myself. My body reflected this neglect. My hips and lower back were tight and painful. I hadn't taken the time to stretch them out, and in turn, I'd stretched myself thin. I was tired, sore, and cranky.

As women, we give so much of ourselves, as wives, mothers, career women, business owners, etc. We are natural givers. It's easy to fall out of balance between giving and receiving.

As women with endometriosis, we go through so much. When you make it through a tremendous amount of pain and somehow end up standing and moving forward, you realize how strong you are. With that strength comes a resolve that you are truly capable of anything.

So many of us push through, never asking for help, because we don't want to be perceived as weak. We can be stubborn — I certainly am. Although I'm not entirely sure where my stubbornness comes from, I suspect it has something to do with deeper issues related to self-protection. Maybe that's true of other stubborn women, as well.

I was notoriously good at giving, but not so much at receiving, and that imbalance affected my energy. Why did I struggle so much in this area? Could it be subconsciously related to pain?

I thought of my own pelvic space and what a struggle it was for me to receive there, be it sexually, or medically from exams and procedures. When my pelvis received, a great deal of pain and discomfort was usually to follow.

With acknowledgement of these messages on receiving, I recognized a pattern I needed to change. I kept the promise to myself to do yoga a couple of times a week, which helped me to get grounded into that root energy, and connect with movement and breath. I took time to rest, restore, and get outside. With nurturing came healthy food, laughter, and fun. I deserved that.

It can be a struggle to take time for yourself and not feel guilty about it, but believe me when I say that you deserve it. Take the time. Slow down. It's Ok if it all doesn't get done. Put joy first. It's Ok to say, "No."

I didn't need to prove my worth or strive not to show weakness. I was strong, there was no doubt about that, but I needed rest. It's not selfish to take care of you. It's necessary. It's Ok to receive help and assistance. You don't have to be strong all the time.

Shortly after my call with Steena, I picked up one of the books she suggested called *Wild Feminine*. The author, Tami Lynn Kent, is a pelvic floor therapist. She helps women release tension in this major muscle that supports your bladder, uterus, and pelvic bowl. It's the strength of your root.

Your pelvic floor muscles play a key role in your overall

support system, sense of relaxation, and ability to experience sexual pleasure. Endometriosis and adhesions can negatively impact the pelvis and pelvic floor muscles. With all the pain that's stimulated in this region, the muscles can tense up and stay that way. Pelvic floor dysfunction (PFD) happens when theses muscles become weak or are too tight. PFD can impact your urinary system, reproductive system, and in some cases your colon. The front of the pelvic floor muscle, near your bladder, is super sensitive, and can become very tense.

One way to release the tension is with a vaginal massage in which you, or a pelvic floor therapist, use one finger to internally stretch, release and relax the muscles in your pelvic floor. Kent reviewed how to do this on yourself in *Wild Feminine*. I felt better knowing how to do it myself. I wasn't ready for someone else to. That felt too personal.

I was reminded of the emotional energy alive in this root part of my body, at the base of the spine. There's power in your pelvic bowl where universal energy meets your female body. It's in this space that you were brought to life.

When you were in your mother's womb, this root part of you was the first part of your body to develop. As you grew up, this emotional storage box filled up with experiences and traumas that were then carried in the walls of your pelvic floor muscles.

Emotions are energy. Unexpressed emotions can gather at your core and become obstacles to energy flow, creating physical tension in your lower belly, vagina, and pelvic muscles. When unacknowledged and unexpressed, this grief gathers. It travels to your pelvic space, suffocating your feminine energy and vital self. That grief shows up physically as symptoms in your pelvic bowl, which then travels to your mind, morphing into mental and emotional patterns.

This area of your body is particularly vulnerable to fear since the base of it contains your root chakra, the energy center that regulates your core identity and sense of security. Fear is at the root, staked in, preventing true freedom.

Another emotion that can easily block up your root is shame. Shame is something I recognized in my own life when it came to my periods and the immense amount of pain that came with them. This unusually excruciating pain was labeled "normal" by those who I turned to for help. For much of my life, the topic of menstruation was taboo, so I didn't really talk about it with anyone other than my mother. Because my suffering was dismissed, and I was unable to discuss it openly, I knew no differently. The pain was my normal.

There was tremendous pain that had happened in my pelvic space, physically and emotionally. When you experience that kind of trauma, it's easy to disconnect and dislike your body. There's a desire for detachment, as a protective response to an overwhelming experience.

Long ago, I tuned out from feeling in this area. When you're severed from your root, then energy is blocked. That pattern diminishes your abundance and causes you to live outside your center. Disconnected.

Wild Feminine helped me to see that reconnection with my root, and acknowledgement of layers of pain that lived there, opened up a path of healing, not only in my body, but also with my soul. When you take a look at this root space you address a spiritual place, though it may be sorely wounded.

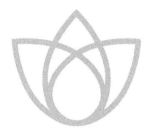

7. Pain

"But pain's like water. It finds a way to push through any seal. There's no way to stop it. Sometimes you have to let yourself sink inside of it before you can learn how to swim to the surface."

~ Kate Kacvinsky, First Comes Love

"How are we ever going to have kids if we never have sex?" Ryan asked. I could sense the frustration in his voice.

My body was tired, sensitive, and sore. Shortly before the question left his mouth, I'd noticed dark spots of blood in my white panties. Great. My period was on its way, which meant three things. One, I wasn't pregnant. Again. Two, pain was on the way. Three, sex was the last thing on my mind.

I'd been two weeks since we'd last had sex. Two. I knew because I kept track. I charted my menstrual cycle. I knew when I ovulated. I knew when we were supposed to have sex if I was going to get pregnant. When Ryan came to me with the words, "We never have sex," I could actually reply with a number of times. Yup. I knew.

And it'd been two weeks. The energy of the house had shifted. The tension was thick. There was more bickering between us. Ryan, like most men, had a healthy appetite for sex. What could be more intimate? It brought connection to our marriage, an intense, spiritual connection of souls.

When that fell away, there was disconnect. I could feel it. We both could. After two weeks I wasn't sure how to approach the subject. There were nods, smiles, and advances, but nothing happened.

One night I got extremely upset. I'd absorbed negative energy from reports in the media. I felt overcome with feelings of hopelessness. My mind went to thoughts of pain, never ending, of violence, hate, and greed. How were we to overcome all this? As an empath, I took it all in and started to cry. It was like a shadow of darkness fell over me.

Ryan gave me a hug, and since there'd been little physical connection in weeks, things started to happen down there. I could... feel it. Maybe sex would make me feel better?

"Do you want a back rub?" he asked.

I nodded, my face still puffed up from fallen tears. The back rub turned into suggestions of other things. While I should have been relaxed, I felt more stressed. My mind started to obsess about the pain sex would bring.

I was days from the start of my period. I could feel it in my body. I placed my palm under my abdomen and felt across, revealing the new line of barbed wire across my belly, stretching right of my belly button across down to my right hip. Things were getting worse. I wasn't recovering as easily after sex, especially near the start of my period. What should have been a time of intimate release, instead just pounded on nerves in my pelvic region making my condition more unbearable.

Tears squirted out of the corner of my eyes. Why was I crying? Again? I feared the pain to come.

Ryan, who was in a different intimate mindset, didn't take this emotional outburst lightly. I should have been moaning for joy, not crying for future pain. The tears stopped things from going further. He left disgruntled and I felt sad and guilty, crying into my pillow.

Truth be told, sex came at a price. An act that was supposed to be the most pleasurable experience caused suffering. My insides took a beating and I certainly felt it. I was left with pain for days. Sometimes there was blood afterwards, and orgasms hurt. It was like a shock wave sent off my nerves, hitting all the endo bumps till my ovary was zapped, my pelvis on fire. Overall, the experience didn't leave me feeling very sexy.

Sex with endometriosis tended to be a touchy subject. I was aware of this from my own experience and from conversing with other endo sisters along the way. It was a big reason why many relationships didn't make it. It's uncomfortable for both parties. It brings a fear of pain and of inflicting pain.

It also brought feelings of guilt, anger, and called into question my role as a woman and wife. What was I worth as a woman who didn't have sex? One who experienced pain with one of life's most pleasurable experiences? A woman who desired, but wasn't able to bear a child?

It takes a different kind of man to stick around in a relationship with a woman who has endometriosis. The sex piece is big, bringing insecurities into the mix on both ends. Not to mention the sexually stimulated media. It coursed subconsciously through my brain. I was boring. When we did have sex, I couldn't do crazy things. It hurt. I couldn't do much that was comfortable. Frustration filtered through my body and mind.

Things got painful prior to ovulation too. The time when sex must happen for pregnancy was uncomfortable, making conception that much more difficult. The whole process of trying to get pregnant was taxing. It turned into a must, instead of a natural flow.

As the tension between Ryan and I thickened, sex turned into a chore. It was the only way that there would be peace in our home again. Which pain was worse? That in my pelvis or that of a grumpy husband? Tough call.

Even though I wasn't feeling great, I decided to sacrifice for the team. The next day sex happened, sort of. Two weeks without maintenance and it didn't take much. The moment came with further frustrations and irritation.

The wells *finally* broke early the next day. I rode the wave and enjoyed the moment, even though I knew it would bring pain later. It was well worth waiting for: an explosion of souls in perfect unison. For me, it was mind over body. I reminded myself that I deserved to feel good. Oxytocin. That, my friends, is a magical ingredient. It calms everything down and makes it all right, at least for a little while.

The amazing orgasm and burst of pleasure also came with pain, and was followed with blood. I shyly wiped it away. I didn't like when Ryan saw it. It was more concerning to him than to me.

Unfortunately, on that day when sex finally returned between Ryan and I, the euphoria dissipated quickly. It didn't take long for things to turn ugly with my uterus. I had an "endo-button" of sorts, a painful patch right under my belly button that started to hurt when menstruation was on its way.

It was a sharp pressure, consistent, and undeniable. Reality hit. The amazing sex had triggered the start of my period.

My lower back ached. The pressure built in my belly.

I started a warm bath. With flow came tears, a deep flood of them. I cried for another cycle down.

Then the anger set in. I was pissed that my period had shown up. I was pissed that after an amazing sexual encounter, I was met with horrible pain. I hated that sex hurt me. I felt disgruntled that I had to deal with his never-ending bullshit. Seriously pissed.

I slipped into the warm bath and sunk down.

Have you been to that place where it feels like nothing can stop the pain? That was the spot I found myself in. Intense stabbing, burning, pressure, nausea, it was in my stomach, and my back. I could barely breathe. Constricting, unyielding torment took me to another level.

There was nothing I could do but be present with it. I felt into the feelings. All of them. Electric shocks of pain. It came with moans and screams. How was I surviving?

It was a complete surrender, falling into black. Maybe like that moment of death when you finally let go — except there wasn't death, no matter the desire. Falling into that place was scary, intense, like being swallowed by a poisonous flower, Little Shop of Horrors style.

As ripples of pain shook my core, I wanted to rip out my uterus. I wanted to die.

What happens when you fall in, when you drop into the darkness of the pain, and feel the sensations as they are? Surprisingly, the intensity of my suffering lessened. Awareness, and acknowledgment of the pain helped calm the current. It took my mind out of the equation. I took away the judgment, I silenced it, and felt how it was in my body.

During those intense moments, I experienced horrible contractions, but in between there were moments of peace— cherished moments. Calm. I savored those moments of relief. Then the nausea kicked in, full force. I couldn't keep anything down, not even water, which my body constantly craved. I was dehydrated, shivering, and convulsing with pain.

Along with the nausea came an upset stomach that caused my insides to pour out of both ends. There was little relief from the pressure. A chorus of hums, moans, sobs, and prayers for help escaped my lips, ringing off the walls of the bathroom tile, and off the water where I submerged my aching abdomen for hours with no relief. Sadness swept over me like a veil. This wasn't going to end.

Once the pain and bleeding accelerated it was as if the prophecy was put in place, a parting of the seas that took me down to a very dark place full of suffering. Was I destined for constant, intolerable pain?

I couldn't help the resounding thought in my mind, *something's wrong*. I hadn't experienced pain that intense in a while. I wondered if a cyst had burst. Maybe it was a sign that the time had come to call for help.

I crawled from the tub to my bed and with shaking hands I filled out a contact form on the website of Dr. Andrew Cook, one of the top endometriosis specialists. I was desperate. I was ready to get cut open. Please take away the pain, the nausea, the dizziness, and weakness. It was too much. Things were getting worse. I could feel it.

My body longed for sleep, but with the terrible stabbing in my uterus, my ovaries, down my legs... sleep was nowhere near. The pain carried well into the quiet night, disrupted by whimpers and continued prayers for relief. I had a meeting scheduled early the next day, adding further stress to the miserable situation. It was the longest day ever.

A woman from Dr. Cook's office called me back a couple days later and left me a message on my phone. I hesitated to return the call. I was feeling much better than I did when I reached out. Now that the beast had settled, was I ready to admit defeat? After my first surgery in 2011, I promised myself that I would do anything and everything to prevent going through that again. The surgery hadn't helped me that much, in fact it felt like it made things worse, and it took a long time for my body to heal after.

Was I ready to go through that again? If I was, it was going to be an excision with one of the best in the world. My first surgery was done via ablation, in which the endometriosis is burned off with a laser, leaving behind the root of the illness. Laparoscopic Excision (LAPEX) allows for endometriosis to be cut out from all areas. Dr. Cook fit my requirements as one of the best LAPEX surgeons anywhere.

As I considered having surgery, again, thoughts of failure rose up, too. I wanted to believe that I could heal myself. I wanted to pass this hope along to others. Was surgery really the way? What extra stress would it bring? These thoughts kept me from returning the call from Dr. Cook's office for several days. When I finally talked to the women who had originally called me, I got an idea of the cost of surgery. The price was as much as I paid for my new car. Wow. That was the price of feeling better? I finally asked for help, only to find that help was out of reach.

Overwhelm boiled inside me. The shockwaves of trauma from the excruciating start of my last period left me fearful of that experience repeating. The pain wasn't easily forgotten. It shook me up. Tears formed and fell as I expelled grief from my pelvic space, sending heavy vibrations into my heart space.

My desperation was echoed from other endo sisters in my support network. Many women felt similarly. I picked up on the fear. I pulled it all in, and along with that came darkness. I couldn't see a way out.

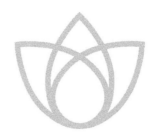

8. Wild Woman

"Through music, which vibrates the sternum, excites the heart;
it comes through the drum, the whistle, the call and the cry.
It comes through the written and spoken word; sometimes a word,
a sentence or a poem or a story, is so resonant, so right, it causes
us to remember, at least for an instant, what substances we are
really made from, and where is our true home."

~ Dr. Clarissa Pinkola Estes, Women Who Run with the Wolves

September ended with a full moon, shining light and shadows through the window. I popped on my headphones and sat back in my papasan chair, letting the meditative music flow through me. The track was called, "the golden way". Behind closed eyes I could see and feel it, pulling at my heart... it was a light that expanded into a fire. I could feel the heat from it. I watched in meditation as that fire transitioned to a dragon, a symbol I'd always been drawn to.

I have a dragon tattooed on my back. It was one of my first. Originally, it was small, appearing not so much of a dragon, but more of a little gecko. Shortly before Ryan and I got married, and I had to stand with my back on display in my white strapless dress, I got my weak little lizard covered up. It grew into a much larger, more colorful serpent, which covered my left shoulder, with flames licking lotus flowers. I wasn't sure why my pull was to the dragon, but it'd always been there. Fire breathing.

The symbol of fire had always been alive in my life. It showed up as a deep terror, and I often wondered why. I had a recurring nightmare of my house burning down, taken over by flames. I lost everything. Then, I'd wake up feeling terrified, not able to fall back asleep. That dream had showed up again and again throughout my life, bridging fear from my subconscious. Other times, in my waking hours, out of nowhere, I'd swear that I could smell smoke. Was something burning? It was an underlying worry that carried with me.

I contemplated this inferno that seemed to be guiding me along, calling forth wisdom. It burned in my dreams, disguised as fear of losing everything, but this was the first time I'd seen it in meditation. My father's last visual memory of his mother came to mind. Fire. I could still feel the pain that came with those past memories, from a forgotten part of my female lineage. There was a deep wound left behind by a woman that I didn't get a chance to know. Were the flames a message from my grandmother? The fire could have been passed through to my subconsciousness as an echo of my father's tears from trauma long ago. Was she lighting my way now? Maybe it was time to finally feel the pain of that loss, and let her go.

I felt a pang in my heart space — I never knew my father's parents. After my grandmother died, a dismantled relationship between my father and grandfather took shape. There was silence, a lost connection to my father's generational line.

I was witness to anger from my father when I was a little girl. It was there, boiling under the surface, waiting to be expressed, appearing in bursts that lived on in my memory. This shifted along the way when he got more involved in the Church. When he made the decision to be a deacon, I saw the light return to his eyes. He'd found something meaningful in his life. Through connection with a higher power, he found his light and shared it with the members of his community, expressing himself as a leader of his faith. He spoke to congregations and found purpose within.

The change I witness in my father served as a reminder that within all the darkness, there's still light. Sometimes you just have to look for it. It showed up for me when I fell silent and reconnected with non-doing through meditation. I got quiet, and connected with my higher Self.

Fire is mentioned in many religions as a source of light, and a symbol of God. In the Buddha's teachings, light is the symbol of truth that dispels the darkness of ignorance. As a flame can be passed from one hand to another, so too can truth.

With my full moon meditation in September, I saw the fire in my mind's eye. It burned with each breath, and as I peeled back the layers, I saw that I was deep in the mud. The darkness had been locked up, buried deep down, living in the roots. I felt my grandmother's energy strong in me, calling me to the light.

I cried under the shadows of the moon, as a greater understanding arose. With such heaviness in my heart, I wept for the loss of this woman I had never met, and grieved the absence of a mother that was part of me.

After the tears stopped falling, I contemplated my next step, and my eyes fell to the book in the stack next to me. It was *Woman Who Run with the Wolves*, by Dr. Clarissa Pinkola Estes.

I remembered Steena's words, "You'll know when the time is right to read it."

I picked up the paperback and leaned back in my papasan chair. Full moon, wolves, it seemed the perfect time. I wiped the remnants of my tears and fell into Dr. Estes' beautifully crafted words.

In the opening pages, she described the personification of the Wild Woman archetype. The Wild Woman is the natural instinctive psyche, the way of women's deepest nature. This wild teacher, mother, and mentor supports your inner and outer lives, no matter what. She's a force within. She's intuitive, a deep listener, and a loyal heart. She is the fundamental Self, the wise and knowing nature. She is whole, the understanding of your soul, and the root of you.

The Wild Woman is the memory of an undeniable connection with unbridled feminine nature, a relationship that may have been forgotten or misunderstood because of neglect, over-domestication, and outside beliefs about a woman's role. This wild nature has been trapped by culture. Not too far back in history, women were silenced and not allowed the same freedom of expression as we are today. Dancing was barely tolerated. Clothing was not to be revealing. I grew up with similar ideas. I wanted to hide my developing body. When I first got boobs, I hid them under baggy sweatshirts. When I did reveal my feminine physique, I quickly got self-conscious. I didn't want to show off. I wanted to be a "good girl" who crossed my legs and played "nice". As women, we've been shaped by a largely unconscious culture that's unaware of this quieted primal force waiting to break free.

What happens when you get disconnected from this wild self? If you believe you are powerless and trained not to consciously connect to what you know is true, then the gifts of your intuition are silenced. You feel lost, depressed, confused, suppressed, without inspiration, without soulfulness, without meaning, stuck, uncreative, compressed, and crazed. You feel powerless, chronically doubtful, unable to follow through or set limits.

That sounded like the characteristics of my early life as a woman, and it described many of the feelings I'd had of late. I could hear the hum of them in reflection of my own life with endo. When you feel like you're always sick, it's easy to pull back from that which you love to do, that which sparks your soul. It was easy to fall into the muck.

Estes helped me to see that sometimes you have to look into the dark to find the light. If you have a deep scar, that's a path back to the Wild Woman. Love nature? That's also a door to her. The sky, the water, and the stars... they're all directing you back to your innate natural essence.

The Wild Woman is present in beautiful moments of nature, in creation, in sights of great beauty. She shows up in the mud, in the roots, in the healing earth under your bare feet, and in the sand between your toes. She can be found when you experience the majestic view in the mountains, or spend time among the trees.

I always felt better in nature, away from technology and Internet connections. I soaked up that time, every minute of it. How often do you fully immerse yourself in the untamed world?

I was reminded of an innate truth that this divine feminine was alive in my energy. Awareness grew from the reminder of this inner light, guiding my way. The fire. The power rising from my solar plexus. It passed through as tears and grief from a mother lost long ago, and followed up with a stirring from the discovery of this inner divine mother. The Wild Woman stirred inside of me.

There was so much that needed to be expressed.

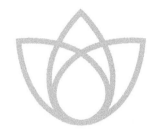

9. Synchronicity

"I choose to present you with guidance that simply reminds you of what you long for most: freedom from fear so you can return to peace. The more you're reminded of what you want, the more you'll embrace your capacity to receive it... the key to receiving spiritual guidance is to be open to receive it."

~ Gabrielle Bernstein, The Universe Has Your Back

October arrived. It took me a long time to be able to appreciate the beauty in the colors of the leaves falling down all around, serving as a visual sign of change. There was a different energy in the air, the light before the darkness of winter. I couldn't help but feel that shift, as if the veil to the unseen was a little thinner. The month ended with Halloween, leading into the day of the dead.

Death. That was my association with this month. October 16th was the day Ryan and I both lost someone we loved. We called it Death Day.

On October 16, 2004 my fiancé at the time, Jeff, was in a fatal car accident. A police officer and a grief counselor came to my door to deliver the news. For whatever reason, I was drawn to Ryan's apartment across the hall. I guess I was searching for confirmation from an outside source that it was not all a dream. It certainly felt that way.

Ryan was good friends with Jeff. The two of them spent hours playing video games and laughing together. I was appreciative of their relationship at the time because it gave me space to study.

One afternoon Jeff brought home a CD full of Ryan's songs.

"He's a really good singer," Jeff said.

I nodded with a knowing smile. There were many occasions when I'd heard Ryan's voice in the hallway that connected our apartments. He sang his soul out for the whole world to hear.

"This is going to be worth money one day," Jeff said, with a big grin.

One night, Jeff convinced Ryan to go night fishing with him at the nearby reservoir.

"It's the best time to catch catfish," Jeff had said, as he gathered up his gear.

Ryan agreed. It was a change of pace from their nights in

front of the TV. They were gone for a couple of hours before Jeff returned empty handed.

"First time fishing together and Ryan caught a big 'ol fish. Me? Nothing," Jeff frowned.

Jeff was out fishing the day that he died. He had crossed over the centerline of a bridge and crashed into an oncoming minivan. His little yellow CRV went right under the bottom of the other vehicle. If that van hadn't been there, he may have gone right over into the river.

After Jeff died, Ryan stepped in and helped me make sense of my new reality. I leaned into that support. His apartment across the hall became an oasis from the grim realities of life after death. The layout was the same as my place, except it faced the opposite direction. It was like walking into an alternate reality.

I sat in a seat that Jeff had sat in for many hours of his life, laughing in unison with Ryan. Jeff's energy was replaced with mine. I hardly knew Ryan, but it felt like we'd known each other forever.

"I had a dream about you the night before Jeff died," Ryan said, "We were sitting together in a blank white room."

Something stirred inside of me when he spoke those words.

"I thought it was weird since we didn't know each other that well..." he paused.

I nodded.

"...and because you're Jeff's girl," he continued.

"Then you came and knocked on my door," his eyes dropped.

"I was excited to show Jeff my guitar. He was such a big supporter of my music," he paused. "He's not going to get to see it."

The energy in the room was heavy with mutual loss. We'd both lost someone who, in a short period of time, had made an impact on our lives.

I didn't want to go back to the dark confines of my apartment across the hall. Ryan sensed that too, and I was grateful when he offered up his couch.

October 16th held another death. Sixteen years prior, Ryan's father had taken his own life. 2004 was the golden anniversary of his death.

Ryan and I now shared a day of loss, which brought us together. Sixteen. Synchronicity. Our lives changed forever the day I knocked on his door.

Jeff's sudden passing shifted my entire world and left me with so many questions. What happens after someone dies? These questions ended up renewing my faith in something higher, and in the existence of energy that's out of sight, but not out of presence.

On that first day of October, I started to read Gabby Bernstein's book, *The Universe Has Your Back*. I read through the first few chapters and felt inspired. I love Gabby's energy. I first listened to her talk during my studies at IIN and I'd followed her on social media since.

As soon as I turned to the first page the message of receiving showed up again, there to remind me of what was missing. Her message was also in line with my intention for *freedom*. All I had to do was be receptive to it.

It was as simple as asking for help. Except that hadn't been so simple for me in the past. I thought I could do most things on my own, that I didn't need help, that I'd figure out a way.

I practiced some of the meditations included in Gabby's book. I'd been feeling out of sorts, not sure what to do, or where to focus my energy. I felt scattered, like my womb.

"Please give me a sign," I said, before closing my eyes and laying back into my papasan chair to meditate. I placed my palms upwards on my thighs, an indication that I was open to receive, and fell into silent meditation.

Later that day I continued to see repeating numbers — 11:11, 1:11, 4:44, 5:55. I'd catch the time at that exact moment. All day long. Repeating numbers are said to have meaning. Some say they're a guiding sign from sources out of sight, such as angels or spirit guides, and that they serve as indicators that you're on the right track, or as reminders to pay attention. After having a strange synchronicity in numbers with death and with my relationship with Ryan, I paid attention to signs like these, especially after asking for one.

As the night wore on, I picked up my guitar in the corner. I brushed off the dust, and went to work tuning the lonely strings. It'd been months since I last touched it. I began to play, feeling the buzz of sound under my fingertips, and as the sound rang out, electric from the amplifier, tears started to stream down my cheeks. I felt a great rush of emotion, as an understanding crept into my consciousness.

It was as if my energy aligned. I felt the shift with the music.

The day Jeff died was the day Ryan bought his first guitar. Shortly after, I also picked up a guitar for the first time. I played for a while, and then stopped. Things that seemed more important distracted me.

Pick up your guitar, Aubree. Ryan's voice rang through my mind. He'd been telling me to do so for over a decade. He kept playing long after I gave it up. His skills advanced to the point that he was composing full songs and playing multiple instruments, but frustration had kicked in. He wanted to play with someone else.

As the tears fell out, dropping on the vibrating guitar strings, it was like I finally heard and understood. I had music running through my body. It was in my blood. My voice, the song in me, it stirred. The Wild Woman was calling.

After the tears dried, a song came out of me. My voice, emotion, and a much greater understanding came to light. Ryan and I needed to come together in music, connecting our energy in a much greater expression.

"Pick up your guitar, Aubree."

I finally heard and comprehended. As this energy and understanding flowed through, I looked up at the clock — 10:16. Was it a sign from those lost nearby? What happened to the energy when one dies? The numbers were relevant. Everything breaks down to zeros and ones — music, code, life, and balance. Sixteen makes up the classic 4/4 timing of musical prose.

As the date rolled closer to the 16th, I spent my time listening to music on YouTube. A recommended video appeared in the corner of my screen, "Run" by Snow Patrol. I stared at the title for a while. I had to brace myself. The song almost always made me cry.

A couple of days after Jeff died, I had a spiritual encounter on the mountain where we often rode our bikes together. It was the first time I'd faced that mountain by myself, and as I turned a bend in the path, a memory surfaced.

On one of Jeff's solo trips along this path, he'd been chased down by a bighorn sheep. He told the story about it often and was so animated in his recollection of the events. I imagined his crooked smile, and the sound of his laughter.

As I flew down the hill, I imagined how I would feel if a bighorn sheep was chasing me. I couldn't help but smile. In fact,

I laughed out loud. It felt good.

When I reached the bottom of the hill, I came across a man walking alone on the other side of the path. He had a big white beard and mustache, and a powerful disposition about him. He sort of glided up the path, in no hurry, enjoying his time amidst the beautiful nature. When I passed by him, he greeted me with a smile.

"See any sheep up on the mountain today?" he asked.

"No. Not today," I said, and broke out into a big grin.

In that moment I knew that everything was going to be okay. Synchronicity. They say it's God's way of being anonymous.

I hooked my bike onto the back of my Civic and as the sun lowered in the sky, I made my way down the mountain. I flipped on the radio and a song came on that I'd never heard before. It was "Run" by Snow Patrol. The man's vocals caught my attention. His tone sent a vibration that spoke to my soul. Haunting.

The words in the song made me feel like Jeff was talking to me through the music, as a reminder that I wasn't alone. He was right beside me. Tears flowed freely for the rest of my drive home.

I continued to hear "Run" on the radio every time I was in the car. I played it at the funeral.

Over the years I'd come across that song at different times and it would always strike a chord in my heart space. That emotional soul memory lived on in the music.

Back in present day October, I hit the play arrow on the YouTube video for "Run" and closed my eyes. As the music swelled the tears were called to life, rolling down my cheeks. I felt the vibration in my chest of loss and profound grief.

Jeff came into my world after a string of abusive relationships. I think his role in my life was to remind me that I could be loved, and that I deserved it.

His death was a major trigger. It showed me how short life is. You never know what may happen. You have to live for now because there may not be a tomorrow. Let go of grudges and resentment. It also made me question what happens after death. Even though Jeff was physically gone, I still very much felt his presence.

After listening to "Run" again, the past trauma stirred up emotions to my chest. The music held strong associations. Music is energy, making it a perfect source for outside energy to communicate. The song spoke to my soul, and reminded me that no matter what I was safe and protected. Light up.

A couple of hours after listening to that song again, I took my wedding ring into the jewelry store to get it cleaned and inspected. Ryan bought me a ring from the same store Jeff had. The man who assisted me at the store set a tablet on the counter and asked my name, so he could look up related purchases. That was when I saw Jeff's name.

"Jeff's no longer there?" the man asked.

"No. He's not," I said. My heart dropped. Seeing his name there was like a digital memory of life passed, but not forgotten.

As I continued to pull in pages from *The Universe Has Your Back*, I absorbed many important lessons, with the primary message being, return to love. Gabby reminded me in perfect timing that love never dies.

The idea of being open to receiving showed up again, too. It brought back to consciousness the truth that I needed to shift and change that energy. It was time. With Gabby's inspiration at hand, I changed my meditation practice. Before I sat down to be still, I made my intention out loud. "I *am* open to receive. I *am* open to receive guidance. I *am* open to receive help. I *am* open to receive love, and abundance."

That was a shift, since generally I wasn't receptive, quite the opposite. I struggled to ask for help, I thought I could do it all, and I had issues delegating tasks, which came from an underlying need for control. I recognized the recurring theme throughout my life. I was always trying to control. It was a shift for me to release, to surrender, to allow and to open up for guidance.

Once I declared that I was open to receive, I took fifteen minutes and meditated. I listened. They say that when you pray that you're speaking to God, to Source, to the universe, to whatever you believe. Speaking out loud your desires. Meditation is when you listen. The silence is where the true answers lie.

When you connect to that space of silence you're connecting to your higher Self, to your soul, and to your innate wisdom. It's the part of you that's directly connected to the divine. It's the part of you that's whole, perfect, and beautiful. When you pause and connect to this higher part of yourself, then you can receive guidance, but only if you're open to it, and paying attention. I think a lot comes through in synchronicity, those little moments that that show up in your life, with meaning and timing too perfect to be coincidences. Things happen at a certain point, at a certain time, and it seems like it was meant to be.

When I opened up, verbally asking, and declaring that I was open for guidance, and I was open to receive, synchronicity did start to happen in my life, quickly, and I was paying attention. Over a short time, I connected with a series of people who shifted my life and perception in profound ways. The messages were clear: there's more than meets the eye. If true healing in my body was to occur, it needed to be addressed on a greater spiritual level.

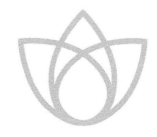

10. Energy

*"Our emotional energy converts into biological matter through
a highly complex process. Just as radio stations operate
according to specific energy wavelengths, each organ and system
in the body is calibrated to absorb and process specific
emotional and psychological energies."*

~ Caroline Myss, Anatomy of the Spirit

I continued to start my mornings with meditation and a dedicated intention, *"I am open to receive. I am open to receive guidance. I am open to receive help. I am open to receive love and abundance."* I took time to listen, and paid attention to the signs and intuitive feelings that came up.

One afternoon in late October, I received a message from my friend, Kristy, telling me to check my email. She'd gifted me a session with a local Reiki practitioner. Kristy had been impressed by the session she had with this woman, and thought that it could benefit me, too.

Kristy and I connected when we studied together at IIN. She was my peer coach, so we helped each other through the program. We'd kept in touch since graduation, and we didn't live too far apart, so we'd meet up every so often to talk health and business.

She was the first person to introduce me to Epsom salt baths, which changed my life, becoming my go-to for pain relief. She was there when I got pregnant for the first time, and by my side again through the miscarriage that followed. I was grateful for her support along the way, and trusted her suggestions, even when it wasn't something I'd tried before, like Reiki. I'd declared that I was open to receiving and it showed up, paid for.

Reiki is an Eastern holistic health tradition that dates back thousands of years. The word Reiki is made up of two Japanese words: Rei, which means "Universal life" and Ki, which means "energy". It's a subtle and effective hands-on form of therapy, whose goal is to restore balance and harmony with your body, mind, emotions, and spirit.

It works through the chakra energy system and meridians, or nadis, in which this vital energy, or chi, flows. A range of healing traditions such as acupuncture, acupressure, massage, and yoga, were founded on this principle of energy meridians.

Reiki raises the vibration in your body, and clears these energetic pathways through placement of hands above or on the body. Your hands are an extension of your heart energy chakra energy, which is where the spiritual part of your being intertwines with the physical. The electromagnetic current that's present within the hands can match frequency of the body (even another body) and vibrate in harmony.

While Reiki is spiritual in nature, it's not a religion. It has no dogma, and there's nothing you must believe in order for it to work, but I do think the results are better if you're open to receiving it.

I wasn't sure what I was getting into, but I was ready to try it. I scheduled an appointment for mid-day on October 22nd. I walked to the small office at the end of the hallway, guided by the smell of burning incense, where a pretty blonde woman greeted me with a smile and a handshake. Her name was Audra, and she invited me to sit in one of the two sling back chairs surrounding a small massage-style table which was covered with a blanket. Soft, meditative music played in the background among flickering candles and a tabletop water fountain.

I told her that Kristy referred me to her. Audra went to IIN too, so we had an immediate connection. She made notes as I explained my healing journey thus far. I told her about the endometriosis, and my quest to manage it holistically.

"I've also struggled with infertility," I said. "I feel like there could be bigger blocks present."

She nodded.

"But who knows, there could be a new life growing in there

right now," I said. I was eight days past ovulation. The timing of sex had been right, and my fertility chart looked good. I'd experienced a dip in temperature that morning. Was it an implantation dip? I was hopeful.

She nodded again with a smile before inviting me to lie down on my back on the massage table in front of us.

"The process can bring up some emotions or thoughts. Pay attention to that, or if you see any colors or have any other experiences," she said.

I nodded in understanding and settled on the massage table. As suggested, I'd removed my shoes and all my jewelry, as the metals could impact the flow of energy. Otherwise I was fully clothed.

"Take a deep breath and relax," Audra said, as she scanned my body. She could immediately tell where I had blocks, and took note on her clipboard.

After her initial scan, she placed her hands around the top of my head holding them there for a while. I resisted the urge to look up at her to see what she was doing. She progressively worked her way down my body, utilizing a series of hand positions that she held in place for several minutes at a time. The hand positions correlated to the energy centers, or chakras, that run up the spine, and the corresponding meridian points. Even though I was on a massage table, it wasn't at all like getting a massage. She didn't rub, knead, squeeze, or press any part of me, but rather placed her hands gently on or near my body. I was very curious about the whole process and stayed aware of any sensations that came up, including a distinct "buzz" on the right side, over my liver.

My energy shifted substantially when she placed her hands near my pelvis. It felt strange to have someone touch there for so long. A ripple of goose bumps took over my arms as a chill passed through. I heard a loud thought in my head, *"I'm ready"*.

Audra placed her hands on my knee and foot, and I became physically aware of this part of my body. Another chilling sensation followed. When she was done, she cracked the blinds and sat down on one of the chairs with her clipboard. I remained flat on my back, feeling a strong pressure at the back of my skull. I couldn't move. I felt paralyzed. It was a strange sensation for sure.

I heard Audra taking handwritten notes, and wondered what she had found. Willing my limbs to move, I finally sat upright on the table.

"You did have several areas of your body where your energy was hot," Audra handed over a diagram with a visual explanation of my energy and where it wasn't flowing through. I had blocks that showed up in my chest, hips and at my knees.

"The spot at your knees was really hot, all the way up to your uterus," she said.

I looked at the blocked areas circled at my knees and saw them for what they were. Protection. That was the gateway to the area that had brought so much pain in my life.

Audra continued, "The pelvic heat means that your body's holding onto different emotions in these areas: guilt, shame, and blame."

I nodded as I bit the inside of my lip.

"Also anger, sorrow, grief, and anxiousness are trapped inside your body."

I felt a stir in my stomach. I certainly wasn't a stranger to these emotions, though they did fall in the list of those that I'd pushed down, instead of feeling through them.

"Ok," I said.

"That makes sense given the nature of endometriosis. It's like a weeping womb," she said.

I took in that analogy, and couldn't help but wonder why. Why was my womb where it wasn't supposed to be?

"Overall through, you're healthy," she said.

"That's good."

I slid off the table, unsure if my legs were going to be able to carry me to the car. Was I going to be able to drive home?

"How are you feeling?" she asked.

"Weird," I said with a laugh.

She smiled back at me.

"Make sure you create space for rest today and drink lots of water," she advised. "When you're drinking the water put love and intention into it to help clear things out," she said.

"Great. Thanks so much," I said. I folded the picture of my chakra energy flow into my oversized satchel and slipped it over my neck. Slowly, I made it out of the office building and stepped out into the sun.

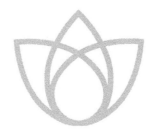

11. Fantastical Kate

*"You're exploring, walking around the space,
but you're a little disconnected from it.
You need to be immersed in the garden of your soul."*

~ Kate Patchett

*A*nother woman who came into my path during the magical month of October was Kate. I had listened to her do a live guided meditation on Facebook within a business-networking group I was part of, and was immediately drawn to her energy. Kate's voice was calming. As she guided the group in meditation, she spun a wooden mallet around her singing bowl. The vibration of sound helped me fall into a super calm state. She walked the group through a visualization that directed the breath through the chakra energy centers. By the end I felt much better.

Kate mentioned how she did the meditations every week in her private Facebook group, which I was quick to join. I became an active member, drawn to Kate's energy like she was a soul sister of sorts. We even had similar features and vocal tone. As a soul coach, fellow empath, and healer, Kate could read other's energy.

Practitioners of energy medicine, like Dr. Caroline Myss, author of *Anatomy of the Spirit*, believe that your energy field contains and reflects your individual energy. Energy data are the emotional, psychological, and spiritual components of a situation in the here and now. Your energy doesn't lie. It states how you feel, and carries literal and symbolic information that intuitives like Myss and Kate can read.

I watched Kate do intuitive energy readings in the group on Facebook Live. She worked within the chakra system to help identify blocks and areas of concern. I watched as she offered clear and honest guidance on how to solve the underlying issues and obstacles that prevented healing.

I was intrigued enough to set up a one-on-one call with her in the first week of November. I went into it seeking advice on my business, but the intake form included a list of questions that got deeper into my health and wellness. I let her know about the endometriosis, and struggle with infertility.

When the call started, Kate invited me to take a couple of long deep breaths into my heart space. I think this was intended to calm us both down. I didn't know what to expect, and was definitely nervous.

"I'll check in with each of my guides to see what information they have for you today, then I'll take a look at your chakra energy," she explained.

"My guides told me to be very distinct and clear with you. Often times things come through as images from a fairy tale or symbolic in nature, or as a song. I'll do my best to translate those for you. Does that make sense? Are you a more practical, direct person?"

"Yes," I said with a laugh, "but I understand metaphors too. I'm feeling very scattered." I continued, "That's why I'm coming to you."

"Without even going deeper with you I can tell there's definitely a lot going on in the sacral chakra region. That's the space that's associated with sexuality, sensuality, creativity, and the connection to your heart space. I also see business stuff in this area: rest and work balance, and the ability to play," she paused.

"That area is blown out on you. Energetically, it looks like a tear," she said.

A visual came to my mind when she said blown out and it made sense. It was sort of like my uterus had blown up. Cells that were similar to those that lined my womb lived outside of it, causing pain and suffering, and webs of scar tissue to grow.

"That usually indicates that there's been some sort of trauma. It could be your body's pain that it has had since twelve years old. I'm not sure if there's something else going on there. I can take a look. I've seen blown out areas before in the sacral and usually it's sexual trauma in this life, but it could be past life stuff. It's a complex space," she said.

"A lot of the time it's the least developed and supported area because sexuality is a taboo topic, and expressing ourselves is another thing," Kate continued.

"I've been feeling stuck and tired. I have a big fear of expression," I admitted.

"Being in touch with your purpose, expressing yourself and your feelings connects to the heart space. It could be heart space issues causing it. Then the root chakra energy supports that. If there are blockages in your root chakra then you're not getting the support through your entire energy system. The sacral space is something we need to focus on right away. You deal with a lot of physical pain that most people don't encounter in their entire life."

I nodded, feeing a pull at my heart from the instant connection I had with this woman.

"There's trauma in that space. Physically and medically," I confirmed.

"I appreciate you being open about it. That will help us get deeper into it," she said.

Kate again invited me to breathe into my heart space, leading me as she called to her spirit guides,

"Put your left hand on your heart and inhale nice and deeply into that chest space. Inhale and exhale, let the air go down through your body through the roots. Breathe intentionally to let the light and air come through in the front and back through your body, releasing out into the earth.

"One more time into the heart space: green, gold, and pink unite earth and sky energy. Expand your ribs, expand your lungs, down your solar plexus, sacral and root spaces. Inhale from the earth, lava fire energy through the root and as you raise your breath all the way up to your crown, breathe out the crown. Open to receiving. Inhale. All the way down.

"We ask our guides to be here today to receive the information that Aubree needs at this time. We are guided and protected. We are safe and supported. We are guarded. Remember your breath. Release any tension. Breathe into the spaces that might ache the most."

Silence followed as Kate tuned in with her first guide,

"You need hugs. A lot of them. I'm seeing an image of you hugging yourself, like self-love, but also from a partner in human connection with skin-to-skin contact. That will help with the lower three chakras. For the sacral chakra try including some movement like gentle dance or hip circles, something that will create some openness for healing, to start the process of healing. Slow movement like Thai chi. Find a way to express that, which is within you. Express your feminine connection, being sensual about it. Allow that to come through and feel it as you do it."

Pauses followed her descriptions as she continually pulled in information from her guides.

"We're going to move to the heart space," she continued.

"My guide here shows me images. She's showing a bunch of flowers, saying to be present in the moment, smell the flowers. That will foster creativity within you. Be more flexible. She's showing a back bend, opening your heart space to the sky. Be more open and vulnerable in your heart space. That may be difficult given what you shared with me.

"She's also showing me a need for connection with your

partner, a head to head meeting, a spiritual desired connection. There's a need for spiritual connection to impact your heart space. Your relationship will become stronger as a result, and help you to heal.

"I'm going to move up now to the throat and third eye. I'm hearing a song... ability to connect, ability to receive divine wisdom from angels, guides, your higher Self. This may mean something to you.

"The good book. It's religious in nature. Genesis. Flowers are flourishing. Things are beginning to grow. You have a sense of a garden around you, but in order for it to grow you have to nurture it. It's a spiritual garden that you need to wake into and hold sacred for yourself. The Tree of Knowledge comes out. You're exploring, walking around the space, but you're a little disconnected from it. You need to be immersed in the garden of your soul."

"Any feedback?" she asked.

It was a lot to take in. My brain tried to process all that she said. The religious symbols... how did it all fit together?

"I relate to what you're saying," I said.

"Nothing's too out there?"

"No."

"Breathe into your heart space, into your throat. Let it flow freely, allowing it to cleanse the spaces, especially in your throat," Kate said.

I did as instructed.

"I'm sensing tension in your heart space. I'm going to explore that first."

She worked me through a visualization exercise of my heart space room — a place of knowledge, wisdom, and understanding. Within it was a central fire all the way from the earth to the sky.

"I'll take a look around with you in the heart space," she said.

I visualized my room with its central fire, a circular space with windows that looked onto a setting sun.

Kate guided me, "Imagine there's a mirror. Look into it and allow the reflection of yourself to show how you view yourself. What might be fully accessible? What you want to change, what you cannot change, but rather accept. Take a look at this person in your safe and sacred heart space. This sacred, emotional, safe place holds deeper knowledge. What do you see here?"

I breathed into this space, taking a look deep inside.

"Come back to the warmth of the central fire, allowing the light to shine in. Illuminate that which is dark to be able to see," she said.

I followed my breath deep into my heart space.

"The mirror is there to help bring understanding to how you view yourself. I took a look in there with you. My reflection may be different from what you see," Kate said. "You're not fully able to be a woman. There's great grief. Your sacral space is blown open, I can see through you to outer space. It's not small. It's big. We need to work on this."

Tears rolled down my cheeks. I did my best to wipe them away with my sleeve, but they didn't stop.

"I took a deeper look into the darker spaces of your heart where the fears and memories linger," Kate informed me. "I asked for clarity on this. What came up was your physical body not being in your control. I saw an image of you being thrown around by your head. You were seven or eight years old and you were dragging this other version of yourself behind you. She didn't look alive. She didn't look dead, but she was very still. You were dragging this other self behind. Not because you want to, but because you have to." Probing, she said to me, "I wonder if your younger self had issues with things. Before you got your period, before you became aware of your sexuality, something that causes you to experience all that pain."

Then she asked, "Did someone put their hands on you when you were a child?"

"Not that I remember," I answered.

"It wasn't in a physical way, but in a controlling way, making sure you did what they wanted."

I paused to remember back to my earlier years of life.

"I have memories of my dad being angry. I have a distinct memory of a road rage incident that happened while I was in the car. My dad yelled at a guy out the window about how bad his driving was, and the guy started to chase us. He got really close to hitting the back of my dad's Corolla. I remember being so scared."

"My dad's mood changed a lot when he got more involved with the Church. He decided to become a deacon, and was ordained the same year I graduated high school," I said.

"The biblical references make sense then," Kate replied.

"I didn't connect with the Church in the way that it was presented to me. It was very fear based. I didn't connect with it. I never got confirmed. I didn't make the choice to be a Catholic," I confided.

She answered back, "I was raised Catholic too."

I felt better when I heard her say that. She understood.

"My wedding was a turning point. I didn't want to get married in the Church. I didn't connect with it. Standing up there because my parents wanted me to, felt like a big, fat lie. That decision caused a break between my parents. I'd disappointed them," I said.

"I was getting images of a father figure, but I have to be so careful in this space. Lots of stuff can come up and I don't want to misinterpret any of it," Kate told me. "Maybe the whole getting thrown around by your head had to do with control over your way of thinking and beliefs?"

I sniffed, as the tears continued to pour in buckets down my cheeks, littering my desktop.

She continued on, "There's a lot of tension in the heart space, which is directly connected to the sacral space. This link comes through in a physical and emotional connection. Physical in the way of hugs, kissing, dancing, and outward expression, and emotional in the feelings that happen within you."

I felt like I had blocks in my heart space because I wasn't writing at the time. I'd been completely stuck. When I didn't write or express myself, I started to feel that tightness inside.

"Let's go back to the sacral space, since that's the main issue," Kate directed.

She worked me through another visualization, traveling in my mind to the sacral space in a tree, anchored with a central fire. This space supported my work, rest, and creativity. Kate invited me to look around to see what came up.

"Remember to breathe into this space," she said.

I did my best to breathe through my stuffy nose. Tension filled my sinuses as tears continued to fall down.

"The same song from before is coming through. It's a Tori Amos song called 'Original Sinsuality'. It came through around the crown, receiving area, and now again in your sacral space. This has to do with sexuality — a sin, but not to you. There's a dichotomy. Is it good or bad?"

Kate invited me to breathe, explaining that there was resistance from both of us on going deeper into this point.

"Sometimes I have to fight through the block or barrier that's there. Breathe into this space more. What's coming through is age 15 or 16. There's another issue in this area. It makes me so anxious," she paused.

I felt the anxiety in my body too.

"Relationship with your naked body?" Kate's words were mumbled, "Viewing it as entrapment, something unsafe, and an enemy to your soul. Emotional trauma can manifest in the physical body. Endometriosis is a result of something that's impacted your body in an intense negative fashion, or it could be emotional, or a mix of the two."

I heard her take a deep breath and the anxiety intensified.

"I'm lingering in this space because it feels like there's a wall up that needs to break down. There's definite protection here," Kate said.

"My first sexual encounter was not good," my voice shook.

"Was that around 15 or 16?"

"I was 17. Fifteen was the age when boys first started to explore down there. It was uncomfortable."

"You don't have to continue if you don't want," Kate said.

No, it's fine. I've been open about this."

"I can sense there's a lot of emotions coming." Kate took a deep breath and invited me to do the same.

I told her about the boy I dated when I was 15. I was in love. He was older than me and had different hopes for the relationship. One Valentine's Day he presented me with a signature pink and white striped box that held a lingerie set, and a box of condoms. His intention was clear. I knew that I wasn't ready for sex, but the pressure was strong. When I didn't advance with it, he moved on to another who would, and I was heartbroken.

What was I worth? I couldn't hold a boyfriend. I was a

beautiful young woman, but I didn't truly know that, or value what that meant. I became attracted to boys who granted me attention, who made me feel good, but I couldn't get away from the sexual advances. It wasn't something I was comfortable with, so I was named a prude. My beliefs about my self-worth further developed around these notions of men, which meant sex, breaking my virginity. What was my value if I didn't? I found out when relationships ended with me, and stayed for girls who were "putting out".

When I was 17, I started hanging out with a guy I met through my best friend's boyfriend. Our interactions pretty much always included alcohol and drugs. One night when the alcohol was running heavy, we made it to his bed. After some kissing, he flipped me onto my back and held his arms on each side of my shoulders so I was locked in, pinned down. He was close, I could smell the alcohol on his breath. His intentions were clear, but I was not ready for more. I was not willing.

He didn't prepare me; he broke into my vagina like an upper cut to my uterus. Rip. He pounded away my virginity. Uninvited.

"I'm not sure I'd call it rape, I definitely wasn't prepared."

"Ten minutes ago, my guide said the word 'rape'," Kate said.

I had a hard time using that word. Hearing it confirmed from Kate made goose bumps rise up my arm.

"There's complex emotions around it, particularly because you feel responsible for your role in it. As soon as you say 'No', it's not Ok," she said, "The guy was not gentle. He raped you."

A shudder passed through me as tears flowed, and my breath caught in my chest.

"It's affecting so much of you: your throat, heart, solar plexus, sacral. You live from your headspace. Your sacral has suffered tremendously." I heard her take a deep breath, and I did the same.

I allowed Kate's words to sink in, and I felt her love on the other end. Truth was, I didn't talk much about my first sexual encounter. I was embarrassed that it happened.

"You said you had painful periods before that age?" she asked.

"Yes."

"There's something else. My guides gave me indication of a past life trauma in which a child was ripped away, unwilling," her voice tapered off, as she considered all that she'd been witness to.

"But the sexual trauma is easily a core thing, given the protection you have. The energy around your sacral space is keeping you from mending and allowing yourself to heal in a deeper way. I can see this around you. You need to let down the walls and allow for healing. You need to receive healing."

Kate walked me through a visualization exercise where I was safe in my bed.

"Anyone who has been with you in an unsafe manner needs to go away. The people who have trespassed. They need to be told by you to leave. Use your voice. Be physical. Allow yourself to win by shoving them out. Shove them out into the abyss. Kick them out.

"There is no need to take responsibility for the actions of others. At the time you didn't have the ability to defend yourself and perhaps at that age you would be afraid of what someone might say or do. That's a normal response. Accept your response as all that you are able to do. You want the people to leave your space because it's impossible for you to heal with them there."

She also walked me through a cord cutting exercise that carved and cut out the pain.

"Release yourself from the memory, from the impact, the

invasion, let it go."

I could no longer see through my tears.

"What has happened in my body, to my body, is not my responsibility. I did what I could. I may not have had the wisdom to know what to do in that time and I forgive myself for having expectations to do better. I love myself. I love myself completely. I am a complete being.

"Bring light in, empowering you. Bring light to the dark holes of this space. Mend the edges. Close the gap. Let it go. Feel the mending light weaving around your energy. Take your power back. Breathe into that sacral chakra space. I am my own master. I control my body. My body is free to be. I am safe. I am safe to express myself sexually. I'm safe to explore myself sexually.

"I am mending my sacral space. I am taking my body back. I've taken the right steps to heal this space. I'll repeat these steps until I feel it solely complete. I allow the healing to do its own work. I receive healing into this womb. I relax this part of my body. I no longer hold the tension. I release the pain. I release the suffering. I love myself."

Then she asked, "How was this exercise for you?"

Kate's beautiful words turned my tears into sobs.

"I can't stop crying," my voice shook with emotion. "I hope that means something's shifting."

"I think you're on your way," Kate said.

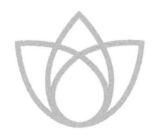

12. Sexuality

*"Unto the woman he said, I will greatly multiple thy sorrow
and thy conception, in sorrow thou shalt bring forth children;
and thy desire shall be to thy husband and he shall rule over thee."*

~ Genesis 3:16

Kate's words lingered with me for days. I was shaken with vivid memories of the past and a strong visual of a blown out sacral space. I ran the images she gave me over in my mind. One in particular bothered me. She described a young seven to eight-year old me, dragging my old self behind, not dead, but barely alive.

I thought back to the time of my younger self. I remembered things being easier back then. It was all about fun and creativity. At seven years old, I was a true Wild Woman. My hair was long, and I didn't like to brush it, so it was sort of all over the place. The Catholic school uniform kept me from standing out too much: plaid skirt, white collar shirt, and saddle shoes. In that sense, I blended right in.

When I was out of school, I ran barefoot races around the house with my older brothers, and sang Debbie Gibson songs in my bedroom. I did solo performances in the backyard with my pink glitter-filled baton. I flipped it in the air as my imaginary audience gasped with delight. I rode my bike and made up adventures in my head. Stories. One of my favorite places to go was the library, which held keys to worlds that came alive in my imagination. I came home with stacks of books with tales from Roald Dahl, C.S. Lewis, and Shel Silverstein. Some of the books I checked out included scripts for plays, from which I selected scenes to act out in my living room.

I crafted my own books with colored drawings and funny stories, piecing the pages together with a hole punch and string. My hand-made books became gifts for my family members at Christmas each year. This hobby advanced, leading me to type up longer stories on the typewriter, producing crooked lines of text, and one of a kind creations.

"We have a writer on our hands," my grandmother said. Every time I handed her something to read, she encouraged me to keep at it.

My mother shared a love for books, too. Sometimes she would read aloud to my brothers and me. One such book I remember was *The Eyes of the Dragon* by Stephen King. My developing mind took in the depiction of princes, evil wizards, and dragons. I fell into the adventure, fascinated by the underlying balance between light and darkness alive in King's words. I was an immediate fan.

On the weekends, the smell of the hot glue gun was common in my home as my mother and grandmother, who were quite crafty, gathered to complete their projects. I joined them, helping create cute little fluffy sheep with pegged legs, and pushing cotton into what would become fat stuffed Santa Clauses with wire-rimmed glasses.

If we weren't together crafting, we were gathering supplies at the craft store. I walked the aisles of fake flowers, ceramic paints, and picture frames, all the while taking in the energy of creativity surrounding me. In the fall, we took trips to gather pinecones that would become festive wreaths. Later, I watched as my mother and grandmother sold their creations at craft shows. I looked up to them for that.

On Saturday evenings we went to church. I liked getting dressed up, and was ever hopeful that after service they'd provide donuts — the anticipation of a treat made the time worthwhile. I stood and sat at the right times during service, but otherwise tuned out the sermon. I did enjoy the music, though. My parents were in the choir and my mother often had solo performances. Her voice filled the sanctuary, leaving me with goose bumps. I looked up to her for that, too.

Once I was old enough, I signed up to be a server at church.

With this position came the responsibility of leading the procession into the worship space with a tall, carved crucifix in my hands, doing my best not to trip in front of the congregation. I also stepped onto the altar and held the book for the priest to read during certain parts of the service. My ability to take on this job was due only to the fact that our church was more progressive than some others. The more traditional ones didn't allow women up on the altar at all.

I listened to the story of creation, of Adam and Eve and the snake. The original sin. I learned about the past blame placed on the first woman and how that choice resulted in great suffering throughout the world. I learned of Heaven and Hell. I watched the reenactment of a brutal crucifixion, and took in the sad face on the Mother Mary statue. I was reminded again and again of sin. There were rules in place; you didn't break them. That was sinful. I was afraid of doing wrong, of being judged in the end, afraid to go to Hell, to burn.

Fire showed up frequently in my dreams. I remembered them because I would be forced awake. My subconscious world was burning around me. I was going to lose everything. When I woke up, I was filled with fear and a heavy sense of dread that made it nearly impossible to fall back asleep.

In addition to the recurring dreams of fire, I struggled with night terrors. There were several instances when I awoke sitting straight up, trembling with horror. Other times I would sleep walk, and wake up in a similar night terror state, often times at the light switch. I was subconsciously moving toward the light, even as the darkness took over my brain.

When I was eight years old, I changed from private to public school. Without the uniform to hide behind, I stood out like a sore thumb. On my first day, I wore a bright green jumper dress over a long sleeve plaid button up shirt, with a belt cinching the center. My feet were dressed in scrunched up socks and brown moccasins, tassels and all. My half-brushed hair framed my face with awkward frizzy waves.

It didn't take long for me to learn that I was different. I went to school in a time of mandatory school busing, which meant that kids were moved out of the schools closest to the neighborhoods they lived in, and into schools all over town. The goal was socioeconomic dispersion, but it also created a racial disparity. As one of the only white kids in the school I was labeled "white girl". There were many days when I ran home with tear-streaked cheeks because of hurtful sneers. All I wanted was for people to like me. Why were they so mean?

I stopped speaking up at school. I didn't share my ideas. I kept things inside, nodding politely, bottled up. The label that followed me: quiet. Even my voice was low. You had to be in tune to hear it, and I didn't share it often, unless by some chance you made it to my inner space. If I let you in. It was easier to be alone because speaking up meant being judged. I was afraid to put my voice out there.

I convinced my parents to let me play violin at school. After much discussion and assurance from me that I would stick with it, they finally agreed. I went with my father downtown to pick one up. The beautifully crafted instrument slipped into a red velvet lined case, shined up and ready to go. I lugged that case with me down the block to school each day. It was worth it for the connection of the buzz of the bow over the strings that I soon learned to develop into melodies.

It also became an artifact for further bullying. Band kids were not cool.

This was the time of my life when my sacral chakra was

developing, and ideas on sexuality and outside relationships took shape. The girls that I hung out with from school were more advanced. This became apparent as I grew older and puberty kicked in. One day after school I was in the bedroom of one of my girlfriends and the subject of kissing came up.

"Have you ever kissed a boy, Aubree?"

I mumbled an unbelievable lie, "Yes."

"Oh yeah? Who?"

Their giggles made my face burn.

This seemingly innocent teasing chipped away at my self-esteem. I was the awkward girl, but I didn't want to be. I wanted to fit in. Those girls began to shape my subconscious understanding of what was valued, and where a woman's value came from: boys.

I'd never been kissed. Who was I? What was I worth? This was a time in my life that I became more aware of my body, and the exchange between male and female.

That carefree girl who felt love and acceptance for my body, and who had a passion for creation, started to dwindle as I developed a new world of beliefs. My creativity shifted to the new goal of finding a boy to grant me that value the giggling girls couldn't stop talking about. I put less focus on endeavors of my mind, and channeled more energy into making myself pretty, so that boys would like me.

When I was nine, I made my move. I picked out a cute Valentine's Day card from the store. It was one of the Hallmark ones with the gold seal on the back, to prove that I was for real. I picked out a red, heart-shaped sucker with streamers coming down and taped it to the front of the envelope. I wrote my crush's name on the front, and slipped it into his Valentine's box, my face as red as the sucker on the front.

On our walk home from school my friend delivered his response, "He thinks you're nice and all, but your head's too big."

She went on to tell me that the other kids wondered if I buffed my shiny forehead. This made her break out into a fit of laughter, and I was completely mortified. I went straight home, grabbed a pair of scissors, and cut some bangs to cover up my tall forehead.

I stopped playing the violin. It was relegated to the corner of the room, collecting dust, the first of many promises broken. Instead of making music, I hung out with my friends at the skating rink, taking in 1990's R&B and spinning lights. Since boys were the big thing, the focus was on getting a boy to pair with during couple's skate.

I saw one that I thought was sort of cute, so I told my friend, and she went to talk to him for me.

I heard him say, "Her? She's like a beanpole."

His comment added further discontentment towards my body. I thought I needed to gain weight, that I was too skinny. The boys were quick to tell me what was wrong with me, and the media was sure to show what an ideal woman should be. Needless to say, I didn't measure up. Next, I worried about my boobs. They were so small. Were they ever going to grow? I ordered some pills from the back of one of my teen magazines that were supposed to make them grow. I'm not sure what was in those pills, but I can still remember the chalky, chocolaty sort of taste. At that time, I was pretty clueless about what I put in and on my body.

Eventually I did find a "boyfriend", although our relationship consisted of an awkward exchange at recess, and a brief gathering after school, before I ran home in avoidance of any kissing. I was terribly embarrassed and not sure what to do.

Going back to that time made the image of me dragging

behind my older Wild Woman self seem much more relevant That carefree part of me was silenced as my attention shifted to external validation.

That awkward preteen phase of development was further disrupted with the start of my period. Horrible pulsing from my uterus made me miss days of school each month. I learned early on that my pelvic space brought pain, and was told over and over again, by people I trusted, that it was a normal part of being a woman. You get cramps with your period. That's what I heard and believed. Except these weren't just any cramps, these were drop to your knees in horrible pain kind of cramps. These were puke all day kind of cramps, as the pressure from a pounding uterus knocks you right in your gut.

That pain shook me to my core. It was traumatic. I'd gone from an active 12-year-old girl, who roughed it with my two older brothers, to the girl who crunched into a ball of pain for days out of each month, missing school, missing fun. My periods were excruciating, but I didn't talk about it to anyone other than my mother.

Pain was all that I knew. I thought that was normal.

I also carried with me a lot of shame around the whole experience. I didn't feel comfortable telling anyone I was bleeding. It was all so gross to me, and I figured others would agree. Many did with snide remarks, or "harmless jokes" from boys who simply didn't understand. I stopped talking about it even though it was there under the surface, a tortured undertaking.

One weekend I was on my period while away at a church retreat. I was so embarrassed that I was bleeding and I didn't want anyone to know. The day was full of activities. When we had breaks and went back to our rooms, I didn't want to grab a pad from my stuff in front of everyone out of fear my secret would be revealed So, I didn't change my pad — all day. I sat in that smelly, soaked pad because of my own shame.

I asked my mother to buy my menstrual pads for me well into my teenage years. When I finally bought my own, I would turn bright red and make sure it wasn't the only item in my cart. I made sure to find a female checker. If only a male was available, I would get so nervous.

I watched as my mother struggled with her uterus, too. I watched as she recovered from a hysterectomy. I couldn't wait to get rid of mine. No more periods? While I was only in the first years of bleeding, I already knew that would be a dream come true. I wasn't connected to the power of that space back then. I longed only for disconnection from it.

I got my first kiss when I was 13. It was sloppy, tongues twisting, face sucking of inexperienced teenage quality. Not as pleasant as I imagined. The fear of kissing advanced to fear of sex, and more so, the fear of getting pregnant. I was deathly worried about becoming a teenage mom. What would become of my life then? What would everyone think?

Growing up in the Church I was taught early about sin and how it related to sexuality. I learned the rules of being a "good girl". Pre-marital sex was a sin, and pregnancy outside of marriage was a sure-fire sign that you were going to ... you know where.

I developed the connection early on that having sex meant you would get pregnant. This belief accentuated when the girls that teased me about kissing boys in elementary school became teenage mothers, and was followed by stories of teenage pregnancy in Degrassi Junior High episodes and MTV's reality show, 16 & Pregnant. There was such shame shed on that. Besides,

I had ambitions to become a journalist, join the city council, and go to law school. A kid would only get in the way of that. I knew that I wasn't ready for sex, but that didn't mean my boyfriends weren't. The pressure was strong. It started at 15 with fingers in my sacral space, a painful, tumbling experience. I couldn't wait till it was over. Ouch. Then it came with gifts of lingerie, and clear signals that it was time for the relationship to advance. When I didn't advance with it, he moved on to another who would.

When I was 17, I started taking birth control pills. They helped with the excruciating pain I was having with my periods, but it came at a price. My mind was altered.

I had little idea of how the pill worked back then. I knew that it kept me from getting pregnant, and it helped the pain I had every month. What I didn't realize at the time was that the birth control pills were numbing me, silencing my intuition, my womanly instincts. The pill does this by messing with the pituitary gland in your brain. This area is also referred to as your third eye, a place of intuition and creativity. I didn't piece together the further decline in my health after I started to take the pill. Nope. I had bigger issues on my mind.

The birth control provided an open invitation for me to officially become an unwed sinner. I was ready to get it over with, to say that I had done it, to prove I wasn't a prude. One of my best friends at the time lost her virginity, and she had lots to tell me about the experience which was all positive.

Unfortunately, the same wasn't true for me.

At 17, my sacral space was violated in a deeply impactful way. The first sexual encounter in my pelvic space was rough and uninvited. Nearly twenty years later, and that act was still strongly impacting my entire energy system. Hearing Kate say it helped me to validate the use of a word I shied away from; I was raped.

The worst part? I went back to that boy, our relationship continued.

Why? That was the question that stirred at my soul. I didn't stop it. I allowed sex to happen again, and again. I thought it was all about his pleasure. There was no attention on me, I was simply an object. I handed my power over to him, disconnecting from it and in turn, my Self was forgotten under the sweat and groans of an animal man. I directed my mind elsewhere, waiting with my eyes squeezed shut until it was over.

He shook out of me, "Nope. You're not allowed to feel good." Those words came out of his mouth, tainted with the smell of alcohol. The devil serpent twisted inside and left me with pain and promised future suffering.

As I learned with my period, I carried forward the notion that sex was painful and not enjoyable. I didn't speak up when the sex left me with blood and a horrible ache for days. I pushed my feelings inside to fester, as the rest of me developed into a woman who failed to see the value in my body. It only brought pain, there was no pleasure, and furthermore, I was a sinner. Sex wasn't supposed to feel good.

I disconnected from my pelvic space, from this center of femininity, housing my reproductive organs. Being on the pill, I disconnected form a normal menstrual cycle. Being undervalued, I disconnected from sex. As I disconnected from that part of me, my creative energy went with it. The creative fire with full esteem, the presence of carefree curiosity so alive in my eight-year-old self as I ran barefoot in the yard, dissipated, a forgotten memory. I was trapped in a body that continued to betray me.

As I thought back to that young woman, I put my arms around myself. You need lots of hugs. Kate's words came to mind.

Especially from yourself, in self-love. I squeezed my arms around that memory of a woman who needed so much love. It wasn't too late to help pull her back out of the shadows.

The darkness of my teenage years reflected outwards in my family environment. My parents witnessed the change in my behavior. I heard their whispers about how I was acting different and their concern over me always sleeping on the couch after school. I was exhausted.

I saw the sadness on my mother's face as I spewed out the truth, "I'd rather hang out with my friends than with you."

The disappointment lines on my father's face were deep when I affirmed a truth I knew would cut him even deeper, "Yes. I'm having sex with my boyfriend."

My father found a beer can in the trunk of my car and threatened to call the police on me. There was a fear of punishment, yet the rebellion in me was not afraid. I was willing to push the limits.

When I was 18, I got a job at Hooter's. It was the first time I'd ever walked in somewhere and was hired on the spot. It made me feel good, validated. I was a Hooter's girl, I was worthy. On my first day I slipped on those signature orange spanker pants over a pair of dark tan pantyhose and waited several minutes before stepping out of the stall. I looked down at the cleavage from my breasts feeling very exposed. What had I gotten myself into?

With a deep breath I pushed open the stall and looked myself over in the mirror. I had a moment of realization; I was going to have to step out into a bar like this, I was going to have to serve food like this. My heart started to pound as a wave of nausea passed through me. Before I could give it any more thought, I hurried out of the bathroom. It was now or never.

The discomfort followed me, along with the eyes of the men in the bar. I was on display for the world to see. I thought that's what I wanted, but in reality, I wanted to run back to that bathroom stall and hide. I tried to distract my mind from the fact that I was half naked parading around a restaurant with drunken dudes who's only intention was to flirt and gawk.

The tempo of the restaurant was quick, so time moved fast. Being my first day, the other servers gifted me with tables that included families with kids. I think they could sense my discomfort, too.

My parents were not happy with my decision to become a Hooter's girl, and they were clear that they did not want me working there. My father was taking classes at the time to be a deacon. What would it say to the leaders of the Church to have a daughter who was only steps away from being a stripper?

I told them I would quit, but I lied. I went back for a second and third day.

On that third day the manager came to talk to me. He told me that I needed to wear more make up, and stick out my chest when I walked. Swing your hips. Flirt with the guests. Lean over. *Give them a nice shot.*

Reality hit. I was a piece of meat, there to make this sleazy guy money. What was I doing? That conversation made me want to run away. I felt sick, used, and slutty.

My parents found out that I lied to them. One of my work nametags fell off in the dryer. It was attached to one of the little tank tops when I washed it. I saw it sitting on my dresser, an open reminder that I'd messed up. Again.

My mother approached me about it and told me that they would not have me living there if I worked at Hooter's. I don't remember hearing why, maybe I didn't want to hear. I was used to giving away my power. I didn't receive the necessary guidance at that point that my body was to be respected and honored, that I was worth so much more. I needed a deeper conversation then, but what I heard was punishment, a threat.

The rebellion in me kicked in.

"Fine," I said through gritted teeth, "I'll move out then."

I packed a bag and jumped into my brown Civic. I didn't make it far. In synchronistic fashion, my car broke down on the side of the road. It completely died. I left it on the side of the road with the emergency flashers on.

I didn't make it to work that day, and without a car it became a much more difficult task. I didn't end up going back to those orange spanker pants. Instead, I begrudgingly moved back home.

I thought back to Kate's question about the relationship I had with my naked body, and how I felt about myself. There was a duality about the subject of sex that showed up: was it good or bad?

"It's a sin, but not to you," Kate had said.

For so long I'd felt pain with sex and related that in a way to my own punishment. There were mixed messages between my inner Wild Woman and this greater pull of patriarchy that was alive in the teachings of the religion I was raised with, the one my father was enveloped in. A woman was to be obedient, sexuality was pushed down and hushed, women were blamed for the sin in the world. After all, Eve ate the apple.

Several times, Kate mentioned the Tree of Knowledge. She also mentioned Genesis, and several times brought up gardens and flowers. All of this got me curious.

I picked up the King James Bible and started reading. I stopped at Genesis 3:16 in the Garden of Eden:

Unto the woman he said, I will greatly multiple they sorrow and thy conception, in sorrow thou shalt bring forth children; and thy desire shall be to thy husband and he shall rule over thee.

I always had issues with the story of Adam and Eve, and the belief that the suffering in this world was the fault of women. My eyes fell on the words *'multiply thy sorrow'* and related to the workings of my weeping womb, to the disease that caused me to feel so much pain. Was it all because I was paying my dues for being a woman?

The line about *'thy husband ruling over thee'* stirred anger inside of me.

Where did that trigger come from? It didn't take too much digging. It was evident in the early parts of my story.

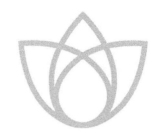

13. Beliefs

"It was in the ashes that she found her phoenix.
And boy it was worth the wait."

~ Rebecca Campbell, Rise Sister Rise

When I was 20, I landed a management job at a lingerie store, which granted me a salary that was enough for me to break free from my parent's house. I split a two-bedroom apartment with another manager.

I spent my working days surrounded by lingerie, a constant reminder of what was considered beautiful and suitable for women — dressing up for sex, presenting your body to the man for his pleasure. This pattern continued in my own life, as I was involved in another not so great relationship. I remained the forgotten one beneath selfish desire. I'd tuned out the act of sex completely.

That relationship came to an end when he spat ugly words in my face, "No one will *ever* love you."

I took those words and internalized them, starting to believe them. Suicidal thoughts rose up. I thought about ways to do it, imagining the slice of a blade across my skin, bleeding out the pain that cultivated in my heart. I cut off communication from almost everyone. I was alone.

I spent nights after work alone in my bedroom, often accompanied by a flood of tears. Not sure what to do with myself, I threw everything I had into my studies. My ultimate goal was to go to law school. I wanted to help the world, protect the earth, and be part of making a change.

My roommate was the one who introduced me to Jeff. Our relationship progressed quickly. We hung out every day. I craved his company. He was funny, polite, and sweet. On top of that, his words made me feel good. He lifted me up, and talked highly of me to his friends and family.

"Aubree's going to change the world," he'd say.

He made me feel loved.

Jeff was a few years older than I was, and worked for a small business that offered tree service. His big broad shoulders and strong chest were stimulated by lifting heavy branches all day, climbing trees, and utilizing a chain saw in mid-air. I liked that he was strong. He made me feel safe.

Jeff opened up my heart again to the possibility of love. I fell, hard.

He was an avid fisherman, and would take me out on his fishing trips around town and up deeper into the mountains. I looked forward to our quiet time by the water. While I wasn't into fishing, I liked being out in nature. I'd usually bring a book or a notepad with me, but sometimes I just sat and soaked up the energy of the river, the sun, and the mountain air.

After only a few months of dating, Jeff and I decided to move in together. It made sense since we were hanging out all the time anyway. We both yearned for more privacy from our roommates. That decision came with a dreaded action, we had to tell my parents.

"We're going to move in together," I declared in their living room.

The energy of the room shifted. The silence that followed spoke volumes. I was going to be living in sin. I was a bad girl.

My father expressed his concern, and my mother chimed in with facts about couples who lived together before marriage and the increase in divorce rates.

Jeff added his voice in the conversation, "I think it's good to live with someone first before you get married. That way you get to know the other person better."

"Well that's not what I believe," my father responded.

Jeff's lips tightened, and I saw my own feelings reflected in his reaction. Quiet down. You're wrong.

The tension remained with my parents as I disregarded their wishes, by moving in with Jeff. Once we were living together, my mother's eyes carried to the single bed in the master bedroom.

"I'm going to be sleeping on the couch," Jeff said, trying to break the mood. Everyone knew he wasn't going to be sleeping on the couch.

I felt like a grown woman. If I wanted to live with my boyfriend I could, right? That's what I told myself, but I couldn't get over the guilt of the situation. I was a sinner. I was letting my parents down.

In hopes of helping to ease some of the stress, and to express his commitment to me, Jeff brought me a promise ring for my 21st birthday. My heart was full, and it was only a matter of time before his promise ring expanded to an engagement ring. He wanted me to be his wife.

Honestly, I was a little unsure. I was only 21 years old. I wasn't ready for marriage, was I? Apprehensive as I was, I knew that I loved him, and that was enough for me to accept the proposal. I was excited to tell my parents about it. See? I wasn't a sinner. Soon we'd be married, and all would be right in the world.

Or would it?

Every relationship has a dark side, and as my relationship with Jeff progressed, it became apparent that ours was no different. Before we met, Jeff told me he had been involved with the wrong crowd and made some bad choices. As a result, he had to spend a good amount of time in jail. He told me about a cellmate of his that became his friend. They still spoke.

This came up as Jeff told me that this old cellmate recently sold him some tools. Jeff took the tools and promised to pay him soon, except the time to come up with the money had expired. His friend was calling him, harassing him for the cash.

This conversation sparked up an argument between Jeff and me. We didn't have any money. I was in between jobs and was freaking out about how I was going to make my car payment, followed by rent.

Jeff had quit his job with the tree company. He didn't get along with his boss and was tired of the way he was treated. He was trying to start up his own tree service business, but he needed basic tools.

"So, you bought a chainsaw off an old buddy you met in jail? Except we don't have any money to pay him. Sweet," my voice dripped with sarcasm.

Our argument got heated and ended with Jeff packing up his clothes into a big duffle bag. He stormed out of the apartment with the bag over his shoulder.

I collapsed into a pool of tears on the couch and listened through my sobs as Jeff tried to start up his old Ford truck. It squealed in protest over and over again. I waited to hear it turn over with a bang, but that never happened.

Instead I heard footsteps come up the steps. Jeff appeared in the doorway without his bag of clothes. He muttered an apology, and sank next to me on the couch as we figured out where we were going to get the cash to pay for the tools.

The next morning Jeff went to grab the bag of clothes out of the back of the truck, but it wasn't there. He stomped around the apartment, his face red, his words threatening.

"He took my stuff," he accused. His energy made me nervous.

"Are you sure? Could you call him?"

"That son of a bitch took my stuff!" he screamed.

I could hear Jeff's angry voice on the phone in the other room before he stomped out with a slip of paper in hand, "I've got the address. Let's go get my stuff," he said, his eyes blazing.

"I can drive," I offered. I didn't feel safe when Jeff drove. He liked to move fast, and his aggressive driving was only made worse by his attitude. What I saw then was not something I wanted to see behind the wheel.

I tried to calm him down on our drive. We ended up at a strip building that looked relatively deserted. The situation made me anxious. I parked next to another small car and cut the ignition, clutching my purse close to me.

Jeff burst out of the car and disappeared into the door of one of the businesses. I tapped my foot up and down, biting the inside of my lower lip. I checked the rear-view mirrors often to make sure we were alone.

I jumped when the car door opened, and Jeff reached into the glove compartment to retrieve the knife he used for fishing. The gleam of the blade made my mouth drop open in protest. Before I could get a word out, he extracted the blade, slashing it across the tire of the small car next to us, and then hurried back to our car.

"Go! Go! Go!" He yelled.

I tried to start the car, but it stalled. My hands were shaking as I tried to re-start it.

"Why did you do that?" I yelled.

Before I could slip the clutch back into reverse, I saw a man charge out of the business doors. He was tall, like professional basketball player tall. I watched in horror as he took a running jump onto the hood of my Civic, followed by a two-foot jump into the windshield. The glass fractured into a ton of little pieces in front of us. With grace on our side, it didn't fully shatter.

Both parties ended up calling the police and it came down to my witness account. One of the police officers pulled me away, and asked me what I saw. I hesitated. My words could send Jeff to jail. My fiancé.

I took a deep breath, my words coming out shaky as I told the officer what I witnessed. Jeff started it. He sliced the tire.

I felt like I was in a dream. How did I get myself here?

Jeff walked away with a ticket and his old cellmate was hauled off in the back of a police car. The damage done to the hood of my car was enough for felony charges, and I made the call for that to happen.

While any day is a bad day to have your windshield kicked in, the events fell at a truly inopportune time. Jeff was scheduled to attend a rehearsal dinner that evening for his best friend's wedding, and was staying the night at a hotel where it was all going down. Since I wasn't part of the wedding party, I wasn't invited.

The shadows of the late afternoon sun reminded me that I was going to have to spend the night alone. A chill broke through me. That man. He knew where I lived. What if he got out and came after me?

Those thoughts took over my mind as I watched Jeff walk out the door that evening. So much for feeling safe.

In anticipation of the upcoming wedding day, my mother and I went dress shopping. We sorted through aisles of plastic covered gowns in search of the perfect one. I was strapped and fastened into different designs until I found the dress. It was a beautiful white beaded gown with satin straps and a dramatic train.

I had images of the perfect setting, a classic cathedral church with tall windows and a long aisle, which would allow that train to expand. I spent what free time I had checking out churches, in search of the one in my imagination.

I found it where I didn't expect to. It was on the corner of my college campus downtown. The architecture of the church was amazing, and the grounds were perfect. I imagined the procession leading down the steps, and the great picture we would capture there. When I walked into the worship space my heart fluttered in confirmation. This was it. The dramatic curved archways carved the ceiling and the circle of light at the top shown down in pure perfection. I imagined myself stepping up to become a wife.

The thought made my stomach churn. I loved the thought of a wedding, but what about the rest of it? Was I ready to be a wife? Was Jeff the one? I looked up to see a carved crucifix hanging at the end of the aisle, behind the altar, for all to see, a reminder of a life sacrificed for sin.

They say once you fall into the system it's hard to get out. That was the case with Jeff. He missed one of his court dates and ended up with a warrant out for his arrest. When he did show up for court, they arrested him on the spot. I watched the handcuffs take shape to his wrists, and looked up helplessly as they took him away.

I had a crash course on what do when your loved one is taken to jail. Number one: find a bondsman to bond them out. In my case, it was a bondswoman who answered the call. Shirley's raspy voice on the other end of the line was curt.

"I'll meet you in front of the jail in two hours," she said.

When she was done, she handed me one of her business cards, held between the tips of her long, fake, red finger nails.

"We'll be in touch," Shirley assured.

The bond got Jeff out for the moment, but the final outcome was a sentence of 30 days in jail. He had a date when he had to show up and surrender himself to fulfill the time.

"I don't want to go to jail," Jeff said with fear in his eyes.

The date loomed over our lives like a black cloud.

The stress filtered through our home, accelerating the energy into screaming matches with each other. During one of those fights, Jeff said something that triggered me, and I slapped him across the face. The shock from my action silenced our voices. We were left with only an echo of the sound of skin on skin.

When the morning sun rose, there were apologies and regret. I had to go to school that day. It was the first day on my path to earning my master's degree. As I sorted out what I was going to wear, Jeff appeared at the closet door. He had his backpack on his arm, and his fishing vest around his chest.

He gave me his crooked smile. "I'm going to go fishing while you're at school," he said.

I nodded in acknowledgment, and under the doorway I gave him a final kiss goodbye.

As the story has already been told, Jeff died in a car crash when I was 22 years old. It devastated me.

I woke up the morning after his death in my parent's guest room. It took me a moment to register my surroundings and why I was there. I hadn't slept much. My dreams took me through the many emotions going on in my mind. Jeff was dead. That much was not a dream, even though it felt like it.

My mother cracked open the door and when she saw I was up, opened it fully.

"We're going to church. You should come with us," she said. "Your father's speaking. He's leaving now. We need to go in about an hour. There's food downstairs if you're hungry."

I watched her lips move, but I couldn't do much beyond stare.

Jeff was dead. The thought resounded in my head. I looked down at my engagement ring. I took the stone in my fingertips and swayed it side to side.

Jeff was dead.

The ride to the church with my mother was quiet. What do you talk about after someone dies suddenly? What are the words to say? There aren't any. The music from the radio filled the silence.

"This is probably a hard song for you to hear," my mother said. Her hand moved to change the station.

I was not tuned in enough to hear the music. I couldn't turn off the buzz in my head. It was Cher. Do you believe in life after love? I hadn't heard it until she pointed it out. It didn't make me sad. I was numb. I looked at her, but she didn't respond, just changed the station anyway.

The landscape passed by outside the window in a blur. A gloomy day of rain would have fit my mood, but it was a beautiful sunny October morning. It didn't feel right for it to be so bright. My world had shifted, yet the light kept shining, like nothing was different.

I followed my mother into the church where my father served as a deacon. It was more traditionally styled than the ones I grew up in. Tall stained-glass windows dimmed down the light as it shone through into the sanctuary. I watched my mother take a dip of holy water and do a sign of the cross before stepping into the worship space.

I wasn't sure who was operating my body. My brain had partially checked out. I followed my mother to one of the first few rows of the church and took a seat next to her on the hard pew. It had been years since I'd been to mass, but I still knew all the steps. It was ingrained.

My father spoke of me and the great loss I'd experienced. He couldn't help the tears he shed in front of his congregation. What is a father of a daughter who lost the love of her life to do? He asked the congregation to pray for me, and for God to listen.

Silent tears fell down my cheeks. With a spotlight on my sorrow, strangers came up to offer condolences. I nodded politely, and wiped away the trickle of water on my face. When the service was over, my mother suggested I hang around to talk to the priest.

"It might help," she suggested.

Maybe. I did want to find some kind of solace. Church felt like a place I should be after someone died. I had so many questions. What happened after someone lost their life? I'd been taught of Heaven and Hell. Where did Jeff end up?

The priest greeted me and showed me to a small room with a seating area. I sat on the edge of the plaid couch pressing my hands together in my lap. My foot tapped nervously. I wasn't sure why I was sitting across from this man, a stranger. Is this what you were supposed to do after someone died? Consult a man of God?

The priest settled in a chair across from me and asked me about Jeff and his religious beliefs. He told me that Jeff was in the hands of God now, and offered to pray together. The silence that followed was uncomfortable. What was I supposed to be thinking? Was Jeff really okay? I had hoped I'd find comfort, but I didn't. I thanked the priest and turned to leave, without asking the questions that swirled around in my head. My intuition told me I wasn't going to find my answers there.

Jeff's death deepened my curiosity about the afterlife. Even though he was physically gone, I still felt his presence. Where did his energy go? Did it transform to something new? Did it return to a greater whole existence? Did it stick around for a bit, checking in with those it left behind? Or did it return in a new body to try again?

I wasn't so sure it was to a far-off place in the sky, or deep in the ground, as in the stories I heard early in my life. What was beyond what the eye could see?

Jeff's passing lead me to Ryan, who served as a beacon of light across the hall. We shared a mutual loss of someone we both cared for, and a close proximity that made it convenient to hang out. There was an obvious attraction between us. Ryan's blue eyes were intense, and his compassion was true. He understood pain.

We were pulled together through tragedy, on a day of death, on a day when Ryan bought his first guitar. Synchronicity. I was drawn to his energy.

One night when the wine flowed heavy in our veins, our friendship crossed over to a kiss. That kiss exploded a physical connection that'd been brewing for some time. Because he was so attractive, I felt self-conscious about my body. Did I deserve him?

Ryan helped me to see that I was beautiful. He told me these words all the time. My nickname became just that, "beautiful." While I wanted to take those words in as truth, I couldn't silence the nagging voice in the back of my mind that said I wasn't good enough for him.

It wasn't until I met Ryan that I realized sex could feel good, and from that point on I was a changed woman forever. He was slow and gentle with me, and actually cared about how I felt. For the first time in my life, it wasn't all about my partner's pleasure. I'd never had a positive experience, nothing in comparison, even with Jeff, a man from whom I had accepted a marriage proposal. I was still under the impression then that sex meant pain. Jeff hadn't cared about my needs. He was all in for himself.

Orgasm is said to be a spiritual joining, and I felt that with Ryan, completely in tune as two sensitive souls came together in an intimate way. I didn't realize the power of this conjoining until I truly experienced it, and realized that sex could make me feel amazing.

Our relationship quickly moved from confirmed girlfriend status to live-in boyfriend. We moved into a house with a couple of Ryan's friends. While we had separate rooms, Ryan never slept in his bed. Only months before, I had been someone else's fiancé, a someone that even in death, lingered in the background, still very alive in memory and in the workings of a budding relationship. I could tell it bothered Ryan, whether it be guilt or uncertainty, it was evident in that first year of our relationship, as we thrust ourselves into living together, sleeping together, and learning more about each other.

One day, I looked over at Ryan and it finally clicked. It was time, I wanted to marry this man. We'd been together for five years, and I was ready. With that decision came the move to stop the birth control pills. I was 27. It'd been a decade of putting those things in my body and I'd started to question the impact they were having on my mood. I wanted to see what life was like without the added hormones.

I figured once I got off the pill, I would fall pregnant, since that's what was happening with all my friends. It seemed like all their husbands had to do was look at them and they would be pregnant, popping out kids left and right. I thought it should be so easy. Plus, I'd been conditioned; birth control prevents pregnancy. Get off it, get pregnant.

Ryan and I were close to getting married. I felt I could take the risk, telling myself I wouldn't be a total sinner if I didn't actually have the baby before marriage. I breathed a sigh of relief when my period showed each month. Pregnancy didn't happen, but other changes did. As the months without birth control added up, my periods progressively got worse. The pain returned with a vengeance. I prayed it wouldn't show up on our wedding day.

With the wedding came a question of faith. My parents wanted me to follow the traditions of the Church, but that wasn't something I connected with. I wasn't sure I ever had. Maybe subconsciously I was afraid of speaking up. I didn't want to express those thoughts, so I followed through as much as I could. I took the steps, until I managed to break away. The after effects of Jeff's death made me disconnect even further.

It wasn't until years later, when marriage came into play, that the question had to be addressed. The pressure from my parents to marry in the Church was strong, as if I'd never left. It was decided for me from birth. This was who I was "supposed to be."

But it wasn't who I was. I didn't connect with the patriarchal system, the fear, the judgment, and the suppression. I knew I needed to stand up for my truth and my beliefs, but I was scared. So, I avoided the issue for as long as I could before I finally did it. I spoke up. My voice wavered, and I was sick to my stomach, but I spoke up — and it changed my life.

Although at the time it was hard and brought a lot of emotional pain, I did it. I spoke my truth, "I don't want to get married in the Church, because I'm not Catholic."

I made a firm stand and I heard words from my father that still triggered me, "I'm disappointed."

That disappointment stemmed from my clear announcement of who I was.

I spoke my truth, and was told it was wrong.

That discontentment carried into my early years of marriage with Ryan, like a black cloud that met with the continued decline in my health.

"Is the pain progressing?" My gynecologist asked.

"It really hurts."

"You're sure you don't want to get back on the pill?"

I considered it, but something told me to push through. Maybe because I could finally think clearly again. That little voice was my intuition waking up.

I was reminded again and again that painful periods were normal. Other symptoms crept up along with intuitive feelings that things weren't normal. The most concerning symptom was blood after sex. My fear was accentuated with Ryan as a witness, forcing me to continue to seek answers.

Suddenly, my fear of getting pregnant shifted to a greater fear that I may never get pregnant. What was I worth now?

"I always had a feeling you weren't going to be able to have kids," Ryan told me.

He spoke the words in my mind. Hearing them reflected back made my heart break. I was newly married and faced with a disease that could impact my ability to have children. I didn't want to admit that I always had doubts, too. From the start, my uterus caused a tremendous amount of pain. Intuitively I knew that wasn't right.

This all further confirmed the belief that I didn't deserve to feel good. Sex meant pain. Being a woman meant pain.

Once I found out that I had endometriosis, all the swelling in my body made sense. The endo belly, a whole new reason for body shame, was unpredictable and sometimes lasted for days. Often, my belly was swollen enough to look pregnant, another lovely reminder of the ultimate shame. Empty spaces.

During Kate's reading with me she kept hearing the Tori Amos song, *Original Sinsuality*. It came through in my crown and sacral chakras. I listened to the song and read the lyrics. The words at the end set the tears flowing. I was reminded yet again that I was not alone. No matter how dark things got. I was not alone.

Within the lyrics of the song, Amos calls up names from Gnosticism, which I wasn't familiar with. As I looked more into it, I learned that Gnosticism is an ancient religious idea that originated in the first and second century AD. The name came from the Greek word 'gnosis', which translates to "knowledge". In a religious context, gnosis is a mystical understanding based on direct knowledge, and participation with, the divine. With gnosis comes a fuller insight, and an inner knowing. The Gnostic savior, or revealer, discusses information that frees, awakens, and helps you recall who you are.

In her song, Tori Amos mentions Yaldabaoth, the Gnostic creator of God in the Old Testament. She also sings of Sophia, the feminine figure in Gnostic belief. She's analogous to the human soul, but also one of the feminine aspects of God, residing in all of us as a divine spark. She's the mother of wisdom, the female Christ consciousness.

The Bible makes Sophia out to be the devil serpent in the garden that convinced Eve to eat the apple. In the world I was raised in, Eve's decision was marked as a cause behind the suffering in the world. There was a blatant blame and condemnation of the feminine spirit. This belief was further validated in the patriarchal structure of the Church I grew up in and the world around us. That female energy and voice had been silenced in me for years, but as I got more in tune with this new-found feminine spirit, I felt more powerful.

I contemplated all these revelations while sitting outside in the sun. I placed my headphones over my ears, and pushed play on a guided meditation that Kate sent to me. It was her signature tree meditation that worked up through the different chakra points. When I got to the sacral chakra, a powerful wind picked up around me, and a leaf dropped on my face.

The Wild Woman was stirring, and I knew this divine feminine energy was calling to me, ready to show me the way.

14. Release

"Singing can be used in your personal practice to connect the authentic expression of your heart with the power of your throat chakra."

~ Kaia Rae, The Sophia Code

$\mathcal{A}$fter spending a week analyzing the energy that Kate pulled from my spirit, I looked forward to our follow up call. During that time, Kate tuned into my energy and gave me a powerful vision that held strong in my memory. I was sitting at a big conference table with a bunch of papers around. She told me there was a guide with me. He was male, tall, and bluish in color. He rolled up a silver ball that lit up.

"Are you going to take it?" he asked.

When I opened up the ball it was glowing. Energy danced out of it and turned into a dragon. The dragon was all encompassing, very powerful, the highest of all animal guides.

My guide rolled me all the wisdom, and I was writing it out. The dragon danced across the pages, so many pages.

"Let it be light. Let it be joyous. Let it be highly energetic," Kate said.

The inner dragon spirit came through, and it's going to speak to the masses. It's what the people will understand and latch onto.

"You have to take it. Step into it fully. Don't look back at fears. No. Keep going. You know what you're doing. Don't give energy to the fear. Are you going to open this gift I've given you?" Kate said.

This visual blew me away. I've always been drawn to dragons, enough to have one drawn on my body. Was there a reason why I'd always been drawn to the dragon? The fire. It showed up again, stirring my soul as it danced across the pages that you read now.

I went in for a second Reiki session a couple of days later, armed with greater knowledge about what was going on with my energy. I told Audra about my sessions with Kate and all that had come up.

"I've had sexual trauma in my pelvic space and she said that's impacting everything, especially my heart space. Those are two areas that really need attention right now," I said.

"Are you ready to release that which needs to go? Are you open to receiving my help, so I can get rid of it?" she asked.

"Yes," was my answer, without a further thought. I was ready. That was the message I'd heard during my first session with Audra. Now that I had a clear indication that this past trauma was still impacting my energy system, I wanted it out of me, so I could heal and finally move on.

I was ready to let someone in to help with the pain. I opened up to receive it. That verbal confirmation was a strong act of surrender. I was ready to let go. I was ready to relinquish the control it had over me.

Audra invited me up onto the table. I laid face up on the soft blanket and closed my eyes. She scanned my body making note again of the spots that were hot. All of my lower chakras: root, sacral, and solar plexus, were blocked, as were my heart and throat chakras. On top of that, my third eye was weak. The only chakra that was open was my crown, the space right above my head, the energy center connected to the divine. While all my other chakras were closed, I was still open to receiving. I'd continued to set that verbal intention every day for the past several weeks before I meditated.

"Take some long deep breaths. Imagine that your body's sinking into the table," Audra instructed. She placed her hands around my head, keeping them there for several minutes.

I fell into the experience, staying aware of any sensations, emotions, or thoughts that came up during the process. *'I should call my Mom'*, the thought randomly popped into my head.

Audra moved to the lower part of my body, and I felt the same uncomfortable tingling sensation when she placed her hand on my pelvic area and stomach. She moved her hands to my hip, and then to my knee area. I felt the pain in my right hip and lower back rise up. It'd gone from calm to inflamed as I laid there on the table, with her hands upon me.

I opened my eyes and looked up at Audra. Her face was focused, her eyes staring straight ahead. Intense. I closed my eyes again and put focus on that pain I knew all too well. I felt a tingling at her touch, then I felt the energy move from my hip, down my right leg, and out to my feet.

I literally felt the pain leave my body.

When Audra was finished, she opened the blinds to let the light in, and sat down to make notes of what she found, just as she had after our first session. I stayed quiet and still on my back, feeling immensely relaxed. I didn't want to move. I felt the same pressure on the back of my skull, holding me in place.

"How was your experience? Did you notice anything?" Audra asked.

I told her about the sensation I felt in my pelvic region and the pain traveling down my feet.

"There was a densely blocked area in your first, second, and third chakras that initially was very hard for me to get through. At the end, I finally felt something release. It was a dense energy that created pain in the palm of my hand," Audra said.

I made a move to sit up on the table to listen closely to her words. That was the release I felt.

"You had a wall of protection around your sacral region like Fort Knox," Audra said.

Protection. It was the same visual that Kate had given me when she tried to go deeper into my sacral space. I'd built up a wall so that no one could come in. The same dense energy showed from my knees, all the way up to my uterus, a clear signal to stay away. Don't touch me there.

I'd gone in search of blocks, and they showed up clearly. Nothing was getting in.

"That protection comes from your belief systems and feelings of safety and security," Audra said.

I nodded in understanding. Safety and security translated back to fear. It took energy to protect those fears, to create a protective armor, until all my energy was drained into defensive mechanisms. Fear was part of my survival. The idea of letting go brought up feelings of vulnerability, and my fear translated to a shield around my sacral space that was impacting the health of my body.

Where there's fear, there's guilt, which is just as destructive, because it is invalidation of your worth and value. Guilt brings up self-criticism. You can try and suppress it, but if you do, it will only be projected. Guilt emerged in me as self-punishment, a loss of pleasure and joy, and it encouraged me to feel negative things about myself. Physical, chronic dis-ease is riddled with guilt.

I thought back to my conversation with Kate and the references to my religious upbringing. It all fed off guilt and fear. I was becoming aware of this conscious programming, and what I'd accepted as truth. I began to understand why, which was the first step to breaking it all down and letting it go. I needed to break free from the negative programming I'd received from the false beliefs which were showing up as strong protection in my energy.

"It took a lot to break through that. I called out to Archangel Michael to help. He lends support, courage, and confidence to help heal from past experiences, and he's powerful enough to break through that wall you had there," Audra said.

I nodded again, not sure what to say. Archangel Michael? I wasn't sure about all that, but I welcomed what assistance I could in getting rid of the negative energy trapped inside of me.

"I finally broke through at the end and I felt that release too. It was long and dense. I think now that I broke down some of that, I'll have a better chance next time of getting in and releasing what needs to come out."

"That's good," I said.

"I can tell that you're open to receiving given the openness of your crown chakra," she said, and then commented on the way I was dressed. I had on black yoga pants, a navy tank top and a black cardigan.

"People who wear all black are trying to ground themselves," she said.

She confirmed what Kate had told me, too. I wasn't grounded. I lived in my head, not my body. My energy was blocked down in my lower chakras, where the pain resided, while my crown called out to its true connection to the divine. I was open to receiving the healing in my body, but I had to get grounded back in my body to do so.

After the Reiki session I came home and sat outside in the sun. It was a warm November day. I brought along a book to read, and as I scanned the words, something caught my attention in the corner of my eye. I looked up to see a little, shiny, black cricket crawl out from behind a pile of leaves a few feet away from where I sat. I watched as it made its way up over the mountain of leaves, and my eyes stayed with it as it walked towards me, in a straight line.

He stopped right next to my foot, and looked up at me with his antennae twitching. We shared a moment of connection before he hopped away.

That was weird, I thought. It seemed that cricket was on a mission to connect with me. Was it a sign? Audra had just commented on my black, grounded outfit and I couldn't help but notice that little creature wore the same.

My curiosity took me to Google. What did the cricket signify?

The cricket spends its time close to the earth, but it also hops around, and its antennae reach out to sense different things, making it more of a spiritual symbol. These long antennae help them home in on their environment, providing symbolism of sensitivity and intuitiveness. These are high senses that connect to the angels and to the divine. As you develop that connection you can learn to trust your instincts more deeply.

The black cricket could serve as a sign, appearing when grounding is needed. That went in alignment with what I'd just heard from Audra in my Reiki session. I was not grounded. My lower chakras were blocked, yet my crown was wide open.

The cricket is most known for its song. It provides healing energy, often in the form of music. The symbolic value for the cricket is finding your soul song, the music that empowers you to speak your truth with conviction. It's a reminder to listen to the stirrings of your soul and make use of the gift of beauty and creativity. It could indicate a resurgence of your inner voice.

Joy awaits if you use the cricket energy wisely.

That night was anything but joyous. I felt the release Audra had opened up in my sacral space, and tears flowed freely. My pelvic space ached as I physically felt the release of that past trauma. The feelings were vivid, like an upper cut to my uterus.

As a young 17-year-old woman, I didn't process the impacts my first sexual encounter had on my body, mind, or spirit. Instead, I shoved it down and suppressed it for nearly twenty years. While it was released energetically from my body, letting go stirred up a strong wave of emotions in my heart space. Grief, pain, and innocence lost.

I knew that I had to feel all of these emotions in order for this trauma to fully leave me. Emotions are energy. I had to feel to heal. That wasn't easy. I retreated to solitude in the confines of the bare trees and fallen leaves in my backyard, and allowed the tears to flow until my head pounded with pressure.

Ryan came to check on me later in the evening, and I struggled to explain the emotions that overrode my existence. It was a lot to handle at once. I felt a pulsing in my uterus, a reminder of the violation, of the pounding and ripping, of my virginity gone.

I expressed the truth to Ryan, through shudders of pain. I was raped, and worst of all, I went back. The relationship continued. I was ashamed to tell him this, but I did. I spoke the truth.

The tears didn't stop that night.

The next morning, I woke up with incredible soreness in my abdomen and pelvic region. It was similar to the way I felt after doing an intense workout. All of that from energy work? The experience had definitely shifted my perception about the power of it all. What was beyond what the eye could see?

I scrolled through Facebook and spotted a post in Kate's Facebook group that asked what people were reading that helped them to advance spiritually. I came across one title that made me pause: *The Sophia Code.*

Seeing the title of the book got me curious. Sophia. I was drawn to her.

Sophia lives in each of us. She's the one who created life in the darkness of the womb. She comes from the darkness, but is all encompassing, the feminine soul of the world. She's Mother Nature. She is the light.

I downloaded *The Sophia Code* that night. The author, Kaia Ra, claimed she had direct contact with Sophia, and that the words in the book were channeled directly from her. The book's intention is to continue gathering light workers to join Sophia's higher tribe, which is called, "The Sophia Dragon Tribe".

Yes. The dragon showed up again. I couldn't help but smile.

According to Kaia Ra, Sophia assembled the Dragon Tribe to reach the hearts and minds of Her infinite children with the all-loving and empowered message of our original divine nature. Central to the High Council's united voice is Sophia Herself, as the one voice from which all voices and perspectives of that voice rise.

The High Council of the Dragon Tribe is comprised of several Ascended Masters who are ready to guide and mentor you. These powerful figures have shown at different times in history. In Egyptian times as Isis and Hathor, as the Bodhisattva in Buddhism, including the Green Tara and Quan Yin, as Mother Mary and Mary Magdalene in Christianity, and as the White Buffalo Woman in Native American spirituality.

Within *The Sophia Code,* Ra devotes a chapter to each ascended master, and relates initiations to activate the Sophia Code in your genome. Each mentor is assigned a unique code.

Over the next few days, I started to see sequences of two's everywhere; I mean *everywhere* — 2:22, 12:22, 1:22. Then, I read the section in *The Sophia Code* about the Egyptian goddess Hathor, and was immediately drawn to her. For good reason, I think;

Hathor's code is two.

Hathor was a creative genius who reflected love and beauty through sacred dance, music, and singing. She was, and continues to be, a master teacher for those who consciously participate and coexist within simultaneous lifetimes. She passes information between parallel worlds through her heart chakra.

I wrote down a piece from the initiation with Hathor found in *The Sophia Code*. It struck me. Beautiful.

"May the union of your vision and voice be blessed and consecrated for the highest good of all, as you create a new reality through the power of your word."

~ The Sophia Code

I printed those words out, and put them in a black frame next to my desk where I could see them every day. I loved the story of Hathor. As I read of her and her initiation in *The Sophia Code*, I continued to see twos everywhere. She was there to guide me.

Hathor's connection with the throat chakra and the color blue is representative of the divine will for creative expression, clear communication, aligned leadership, self-mastery, revealing truth, and freedom of speech.

And song.

Shortly after I read that passage from Hathor's section in the book, a beautiful song flowed out of me:

> *I see you*
> *Shining in your light,*
> *Even though*
> *You may not see it for yourself.*

Call on me
When you lose your way.
It may be dark,
But the light's inside.

You are part of me,
In your sovereignty.
We will rise above
Once you share your light
And shine, shine out the dark
Shine, shine, shine out the dark.

Don't give up.
We will make it through.
Even through
That may not feel possible now.

All it take's
A little faith.
It may be dark,
But the light's inside.

You are part of me,
In your sovereignty.
We will rise above
Once you share your light
And shine, shine out the dark.
Shine, shine, shine out the dark.

The time is now.
To raise your light.

You are light.
We are light.
Let's raise our light.
Heal the world.

The time has come.
Raise the vibration.
Love and light.

I found myself humming it on my walks with my dogs, and any time I felt the energy of fear. I felt better when I sang it. Safe.

It came from explorations of Sophia, and the love I felt as I read *The Sophia Code*. I believed there was magic being passed to me through those words, and I think it no coincidence that it all came out after Kate's vision of my blue guide, rolling me a silver ball with stars, and the energy of the dragon, the cricket, and of course, the Sophia Dragon Tribe!

I was drawn to Sophia. The divine feminine was not something I grew up with. It was not something I knew of, yet it was providing me with great comfort in a time when I very much needed it. Whether Kaia Ra's words were transcribed directly from Sophia or not, it made no difference to me at the time. When I picked up the book I felt better, and that's what I needed in the moment.

My discovery of Hathor, and my newfound connection to the divine feminine, sparked a reminder of my love for music and for singing. I recognized how healing that alone could be, combining my words and the literal vibration of my throat chakra. Singing was a way to express myself. It was the sound of my soul. It made me think more about this medium of sound and how it was going to play out in my future.

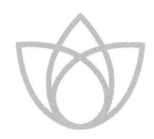

15. Angels

"As you sit there reading this–whether you believe this or not–
there is an angel by your side: it is your guardian angel and
it never leaves you. Each one of us has been given a gift,
a shield made of the energy of light."

~ Lorna Byrne, Angels in My Hair

The connections I'd made in a short period of time with people involved with energy work and Spirit guides intrigued me. What was really beyond what the eye could see? I'd always been drawn to paranormal stories, and held great curiosity for the afterlife and spirits.

For much of my life, I related the unknown to bad things. I'd always had an innate fear of the dark, perhaps because it felt out of control. What was there that I couldn't see? It's within the dark that your other senses heighten, becoming more primal and instinctual. A feeling.

Growing up, there was a long line of stairs leading to the top floor where my bedroom was. I hated walking up that long staircase at night, and I wouldn't do it when there was no one else upstairs. The fear of that dark hallway was almost paralyzing. Mixed with the night terrors that showed up frequently in my sleep, I instinctively moved to the light switch, to turn off the darkness.

I was aware that there was badness out there in the world. Every night before bed I watched as my father made his rounds, locking all the doors in the house and placing a wooden stick into the track of the sliding glass door to prevent anyone opening it from the outside. We were taught to always lock the door because we needed protection from whatever was out there, but could the locks really keep it all away?

When I was 13, I spent my afternoons watching episodes of the soap opera Days of Our Lives. There was a period of time when one of the main characters, Marlena, was possessed by the devil, which, of course, required a dramatic exorcism. The idea of possession by the devil freaked me out. The images from the show stayed in my mind, preventing sleep, until I'd finally drift into disturbing dreams. After that, I avoided watching any shows that included demon possession. That concept really stirred my soul — I was afraid of being taken over by the darkness.

As my teenage years progressed, along with the physical and emotional pain, I did everything I could to create an alternative reality, to escape my body. I chugged Bacardi and lemonade and put mind-altering drugs into my body, including LSD. The last time I tripped on acid, it scared me enough to never do it again.

There was a movie out at the time called *The Devil's Advocate*, which includes a vivid scene that etched itself into my memory. In the film, the wife, Mary Ann, starts to see demons, which drive her crazy until eventually, she slits her own throat. The last time my mind tripped out, the image of that demon showed up on my own face when I looked into the mirror. My altered state allowed me to see a shadow that scared the crap out of me — the demon inside.

Hell played out in my body in the years to come with horrible, unyielding pain that resulted in a barren womb and an aching heart. Why? Was it payment for my sins, or just a part of this life I was given?

While my mind held fear of the dark, I didn't give as much thought to the light. My thoughts on God, angels, and miracles were all parts of stories I heard in church. I'm not sure I gave much weight to them.

Even my soul felt like a foreign concept. The only thought I had of it back then was that it would either go to heaven or to hell. I worried about the dark side, and hoped that I'd done enough to be picked for the good side. The thought worried me for many years; was I good enough?

My perspective shifted profoundly when I realized I could connect with my soul while I was still living here on Earth, in this human experience. I'd discovered this truth because of the darkness. When the pain overtook me, and my knees hit the floor, I was in perfect position to look up. Even through all of it I had to ask: what's the lesson to be learned from this? Why?

My spirit was giving off unspoken signs that an intuitive like Kate could pick up on. I was reflecting pain, sorrow, grief, and moments of joy and creativity, like a soul vibe. These messages of my soul carried deeper meaning; answers to the never-ending question of 'why'. Why the suffering?

I found myself drawn to more women who practiced energy work and greater spiritual understanding that emphasized a close and personal connection with your soul in the present moment. I became fascinated by all of it, especially after experiencing such a physical response to the energy work that was done on me. I was starting to "see" that there was more impacting my physical existence than met the eye.

I'd always been sensitive, intuitive, and empathic. I'd been picking up on energy my entire life, but I wasn't really conscious of it, nor did I understand it, until now. I'd finally opened myself up to receive it, and realized that there was so much that needed to be let go. Emotions are energy in action, but in order for them to pass through, they need to be acknowledged and felt. When they are shoved down, and not felt through, they gather.

Your soul energy doesn't lie. It's made up of your truth. It vibrates at higher frequencies of love, joy, and peace. It's you, true, beautiful, and whole. The light of spirit is stronger than the dark because its existence is made from pure love, and love is greater than fear.

I wanted to connect more to this soul energy, to the real me. That connection had been overshadowed for so long, and it was time for me to finally look toward the light.

My growing connections with other intuitive women, and curiosity about their tactics, led me to pick up my first tarot card deck, followed by my first angel oracle card decks. Honestly, I'd always been afraid of tarot cards. For whatever reason, I related them to witchery and darkness.

Turns out that wasn't true at all. Quite the opposite, actually. The cards served as a spiritual tool to tap into the language of my soul. My emotional state, beliefs, and thoughts were all vibrating out. The cards were an instrument to pick up on my own energy and the messages it gave off, as a reflection of my truth.

The oracle card deck I picked up was from Doreen Virtue, a woman I'd known as "the angel lady." Doreen is a clairvoyant with a background in psychology. Her mother was a Christian spiritual healer and her father was a self-employed writer. Doreen worked as a psychotherapist until her life was saved by divine intervention during an armed carjacking. After this experience she focused solely on researching and teaching about divine intervention.

Oracle cards are an ancient and time-honored way to connect with your angels. They're based upon Pythagorean numerology, which teaches that numbers and images all vibrate in a very precise, mathematical way. They operate within the infallible Law of Attraction. This means your inquiries will always attract the perfect cards as answers; each one you pull will exactly match the vibration of the question.

The box of oracle cards I got from Doreen were of the Angels. Following the instructions on the box, I cleared the cards with a small prayer, and then briefly touched all the cards, introducing my energy to each one.

I asked a question aloud as I shuffled the cards, "What do I need to know today?"

The messages I needed to receive for the day were indicated by any cards that "jumped" out of the deck as I shuffled. Every card was positive, so I didn't need to worry about choosing wrong.

The answers or advice that appeared were right on point, every time. It started to wig me out a bit. I was putting off a vibe that could be counseled by a spiritual part of myself, and the cards served as a way to manifest my intuition. They were in no way connected to darkness. They were simply a tool which allowed access to messages of healing and self-discovery for the explorative part of me that sought answers, especially as I came closer to my 35th birthday, the age I'd been dreading for so long.

I saw Audra a few days before my birthday. She smiled when I told her about the nearly pain-free period I'd experienced. I told her about the book *Medical Medium*, and the success I'd had with implementing his suggestions, especially the addition of fresh organic celery juice to my morning routine.

"The celery juice helps strengthen your stomach acid," I explained. "So, it strengthens your digestion and immune system overall. I've been feeling much better since starting my day with the celery juice. Things are flowing out," I laughed.

This branched out to further conversation about the author, Anthony William, his connection to Spirit, and his ability to help people with chronic conditions.

"There's another book I recommend you read called *Angels in My Hair*, by Lorna Byrne. She completely changed my perspective on things," Audra said.

I made a note to pick up the book, as I slipped off my shoes and jewelry. I settled back on the treatment table as usual, and closed my eyes. Audra scanned my body making note of the chakra areas that were blocked, including my root chakra.

"Your hips are much better," she told me.

Once she did her initial scan, she went through the now familiar routine, placing her hands on top of my head as I took a series of long deep breaths and tuned into my sensations. She moved down my body until she reached my sacral space. As she placed her hands near my pelvis her touch was steady, but it felt heavy, like she was going deeper in. I felt a tingling in my third eye.

Pictures flashed in my mind. First, the face of the man who stole my virginity from me, then, another man's face. He was older and oddly familiar, though I couldn't put my finger on why I knew him. It was as if he was looking at me, hovering over my consciousness. I didn't sense any negative energy from him, more like a feeling that I was safe now. He was watching me.

I felt a release from deep in my pelvis. Even after Audra moved her hands away, it felt like she was still touching me. There was a heavy presence on my right side. When she was done with the session, Audra opened the blinds and allowed the light to shine in the room. I felt the familiar pressure on the back of my head as I laid still on the table. My mind swirled with a single thought — *who was that man?*

Audra broke the silence, "I could easily access your sacral space this time. The walls have dropped. It felt like I got out all the blocked energy from the region in your hip and lower back."

"That's good," I said, as I slowly moved to sit up.

"We'll know more next time I see you," she assured me with a smile.

I nodded, still in a daze.

When I came home, I couldn't stop thinking about the image of the face I'd seen so clearly. Who was he? I brought up the experience to Ryan, amidst the fear that he would think I was a crazy person. He listened to me, and along with me, had hope that maybe some deeper healing was happening. Even though my scientific brain could not fully explain it, a deeper part of myself knew something had shifted.

My birthday came and went. Life went on at 35.

I pulled out the Christmas decorations and prepared my front room for the coming festivities. Originally, I wasn't going to decorate, but I'd changed my mind. It didn't feel right being in the holiday season without the twinkling lights of the tree.

As I unpacked the boxes, I couldn't help but notice how many angels there were. Every year my mother bought me an ornament for the tree, and most years mine was an angel. They surrounded the tree. I pulled open a box with one that she'd gifted me the year before.

The head had gotten separated from the body. I got a feeling in my belly as I took in the image of this small headless creature. It didn't seem right to see a decapitated angel. I lifted the detached piece, and looked into the blue eyes of the light-haired figure. It was then I noticed some roman numerals carved on it. I jotted them down on a piece of paper, so I could translate them. It was a date: 1998.

I thought back to December of that year. I turned 17. The decapitated angel was inscribed with the year that my virginity was lost, by violation. How appropriate; that's when I began to disconnect my head from my body.

I popped the disconnected appendage into place, and looked at the figure in front of me. Now, she was complete.

I ordered the book that Audra recommended to me: *Angels in My Hair*, by Lorna Byrne, and spent the following weekend consuming the story of this Irish mystic that could see and communicate with angels. She'd been doing so since she was a baby. The book was the first time she'd come out publicly with her experience of what she'd seen and learned.

Lorna claimed that your guardian angel's always there, but in order to receive its help, you have to ask. There are so many angels lingering about waiting to help, except most people don't believe in them, so they don't talk to them, and the guardians are left waiting and hoping to be of assistance.

By asking them to help you, you make a stronger connection with your angel and those around you.

Lorna's story changed my perspective, too. It was comforting to me to believe that there was love and protection around me all the time. I was loved, and when I spoke up, my voice was heard.

I shifted my prayers to addressing the angels, and found that many of them were granted. I called upon them in situations that felt out of control. I asked for their protection and love for myself and my loved ones. I visualized their love and light around me. I was safe.

I know for some this may be hard to believe. It's easy to be a skeptic when something's beyond what your eyes can see, much like the disbelief that comes from people when you have an invisible illness, like endometriosis.

What does it hurt to consider the possibility? What do you have to lose by opening up your spiritual self, and learning about your soul? Ask your angel to help you, now. They're ready to support and guide you.

You're not alone. You'll never be alone. Even in the darkest hour, there's light all around, waiting to be called upon. You simply have to speak up, ask, and be open to receive.

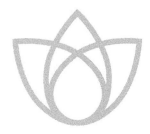

16. Expression

*"Maybe you are searching among the branches
for what appears only in the roots."*

~ Rumi

*I*t felt like synchronistic messages were driving me to speak out, fueled by a rising Wild Woman inside, the divine feminine, Sophia, Hathor. I needed to express myself. I visualized a future with me up on stage, using my voice, helping other women to find peace.

The visual shouldn't have come as a huge surprise to me, as the practice was rooted in my family. My mother showed this to me as a child, singing out her voice into the church, and later my father took the stage as a spiritual leader. I sought to be a facilitator and leader within a group of women who've been silenced for far too long. I'd shaped myself into a voice for those living with endometriosis.

As the end of the year approached, I gifted myself two things. One was a Blue Yeti microphone. I decided to capture my voice and share it with the world by starting a podcast. I've always been drawn to music, to sound. When I was younger, one of my dreams was to become a radio DJ. What a great job, to sit around and listen to music all day. The podcast seemed like a natural manifestation of my youthful career fantasies.

The other gift I gave to myself was a Himalayan singing bowl. I'd done some meditations where one was used, and I found it to be super relaxing. I didn't know much about singing bowls when I bought one, but later learned that the sound of the singing bowl is at a different vibration, and some say it's the sound of your soul.

The bowl brought an amazing new vibrational element to my day. The rhythm of my hand spinning in a symbolic circle of life, caused the bowl to ring out soothing waves of sound. Whenever I was feeling out of sorts, I sat down and got grounded.

I unpacked my Blue Yeti microphone and set it up on my desk. I felt like the real deal. Peace with Endo would be the name, and I relayed my excitement about my new podcast on social media to pump up the momentum for its release. Yet, behind the scenes, I was afraid.

I found myself drowning in a list of excuses for why it wasn't getting done. Weeks passed. I had an episode recorded, but I overanalyzed it. Then I let Ryan listen to it with his keen musician ears, and became even more aware of the imperfections. I re-recorded it again, and again.

Eventually, I reached a point when I thought it sounded good and was ready to be released to the world. That day was Valentine's Day, the day of love, heart, and connection. How perfect.

Every year my father sends a card postmarked from Loveland, Colorado. I picked up my phone to call and thank him. Our conversation was short and to the point, with a quick exchange of love and gratitude.

Before the call disconnected, my mother got on the line. We chatted for a bit, and I told her about the release of my new podcast. She had recently gotten into listening to podcasts on the way to work.

"I'll be listening," she said.

After I hung up the phone, her words stayed with me. The perfectionist in me stirred up. I re-listened to the episode multiple times, and over evaluated it. Knowing that my mother was going to be listening sparked up worry. What would she think?

I went to grab my laptop and to listen yet again, but before I got there, I tripped over the cord to the headphones. My breath caught as the cord pulled from the computer with the jack still in the input, breaking in the process.

A little while after that incident, I had a call with Kate. I wanted to check in on the progress with my energy since the intense Reiki session I had with Audra, and also to gain guidance on how I could be of service to the endometriosis community. Every day I connected with women who were struggling with pain both physically and emotionally. What could I do to help alleviate that?

I'd struggled for years to remove the pain with my periods, and after experiencing energy work I'd had three cycles in a row with little to no pain. I didn't have much cramping leading up to my period, and felt better overall than I normally did. When my period arrived, I waited for the pain. There was a little cramping, but I found relief fairly quickly after a warm bath with Epsom salt. I waited for the trauma to ensue, for the horrible cramps and contractions to come, but they didn't. I felt strangely fine.

This made me more curious about the role of energy and its connection with endometriosis. How could I help share the success I was experiencing with other endo sisters?

As Kate tuned into my energy, she asked how the spiritual aspect was feeling in my life.

"Good," I said after a moments pause. "That part feels strong."

"I asked because your crown space is totally open. Not everyone's experience is like that."

I told Kate about my new intention setting before meditation. I *am* open to receive. I *am* open to receive love and abundance. I *am* open to receive help. I *am* open for guidance. Ever since doing that, I was divinely guided to the information that I needed to know. It brought me to Kate.

"I've been more open to angels, which wasn't something that I'd really considered before. They've always been these mystical beings. Have you heard of Lorna Byrne?"

"I have," Kate said.

"Her book *Angels in My Hair* totally changed my perspective. I've shifted my prayers to the angels, to asking for help, and more things have been happening since then." I thought back to all the magical synchronicity that had shown up, and the messages I'd been reviewing in subtle hints and nudges.

"I can tell that the spiritual aspect is strong because your crown is wide open. The areas that need to be addressed are in your root and throat chakras. Your root is what connects your body to your soul. It's the earth energy that you always have access to. The spiritual and emotional connection in the root energy connects to the rest of you," Kate said.

We both directed our attention to the root chakra space in my body. What she said next stirred my soul.

"You've staked yourself in the ground, putting a nail through your foot to keep yourself steady and anchored. It's a forced grounding. It's as if your soul is wanting to escape your body. You're living in your head space, not in your body," she said.

I'd felt the desire for escape, to fly away from this shell of a body that brought so much pain. It'd been a pattern of mine for most of my life to want to run away from it in some way or another.

"There is fear here. A sense of lack, not having enough to sustain," Kate continued, as she explored more of my root. "Your root space is craving spiritual connection with others. You're looking around and wondering, *Why am I doing this by myself?* It's a lonely and isolated feeling."

I felt the tears start to rise up. Kate had a way of picking up on all the emotions gathered there, silent, unexpressed. She pulled them out to be recognized. Kate moved up into my sacral space to explore again this idea of sexuality.

"I saw you laying down and scanning yourself, paying close attention to how your body feels. You're looking at it like a medical experience and not spiritual, or something where you feel emotions. You're scanning your body for trouble. It's a thing to be watched, rather than something to experience joy. It's like you're walking away from that connection.

"It's a spiritual disassociation from your body in terms of sexuality. So, you're improving it in a medical sense, rather than seeing it as a sensual, sexual being. Your body is doing Ok, but you're not allowing your soul to infuse into your body space," Kate said.

She recommended that I continue to work on grounding myself, and as I'd been setting an intention to be open to receiving, I also needed to be open in my root, to allow the mother earth goddess, divine feminine, to flow into my lower body. I could connect my breath and body into soul energy.

"I don't feel grounded. It's like I'm floating around," I told her. I was living in my headspace.

My sacral chakra echoed the root.

"You're spinning in circles energetically. Searching, searching, searching, looking outside, when the answer is within. There's a body disconnect. It's very uncomfortable in the physical and there's a strong desire to escape."

The same theme showed up in my heart space. I didn't want to deal with whatever was going on there, which was causing my energy to leave my body, floating out in space, totally out of body sometimes. This area was heavily protected. Kate picked up images of a tiger and leopard.

"Let's move to the throat space. Energetically, it has been throbbing. If we take care of this the other things will be helped.

Your throat chakra connects with truth, visibility, the ability to hear the truth from others, and communication from them. It is here where you can manifest things you receive through Spirit and how you express yourself," Kate said.

She paused as she tuned into my throat chakra.

"Things are clogged here in body and mind. It's foggy and hard to see," Kate said with a deep breath.

"You say, 'I've lit my lamp. I'm standing my ground. I know my message,' yet you're being very guarded. Self-judging. Wanting to do the best, wanting to be very good at what you're doing and afraid of how people perceive that. You're judging yourself before they even could, and it's making you at a standstill. There's protection here.

"I see you being held by your hand then pulled back really quick and admonished. You're very sad after that. The throat issue is impacting your third eye. The third eye and throat are connected. This is impacting your abilities to bring messages from source, from your higher Self, your divine purpose through your physical body. It gets muddled. It's clogged up in there."

I listened to Kate's accounts in awe. She had picked up on the fear I felt about releasing the podcast out into the world, and the judgment I'd placed on myself.

Kate continued, "You wonder, 'How can my one point of light matter?' It's foggy in here. There's definitely a lot going on in the throat space."

I filled in Kate on my intention to start the *Peace with Endo Podcast.*

"The first episode has been done for about a month, but I've had fear of putting it out there. It's dipping more into the spiritual side of things. I got the episode ready, and I was going to publish it, to get it out into the world, then I talked to my mom on Valentine's Day."

The conversation with my mother had triggered something in me. I'll be listening. Perfectionist tendencies rose up. I held a fear of being judged about speaking on spiritual matters that were somewhat outside of what I'd grown up with. I was curious about many things, and my conversations with Kate only confirmed that there was definitely more than met the eye.

I felt anxious after that conversation that I had with my mother. A resounding thought sounded through, *I'm not enough.* That thought pattern drove me to re-listen to my recording ten more times. It made me overanalyze every last breath.

I told Kate about my headphones, how I'd tripped over the cord.

"I think it was a sign. I need to cut the cord," I said.

Kate agreed.

"Are you ready to do that?" she asked.

"Yes," I said with certainty.

Kate invited me to breathe white protective light into my heart space and to exhale it out, with my mouth open, releasing the fogginess in my throat space.

She confirmed that my truth had been suppressed. Somewhere along the line I was told I was wrong for doing or saying something. Someone yanked my hand, pulling me away so that I wouldn't say or do whatever it was, and it crushed my heart.

"No. That's not right. That's wrong," Kate said.

I had a cord in my throat and heart space that was connected to my mother and keeping tabs. It was controlling my throat space to a certain extent. It was time to cut that loose.

"It's very complex in there," Kate said.

I felt through the emotions and feelings that coursed in my

body. Tears stirred again, catching in the back of my throat.

"We'll send the energy back to her with love and compassion. Anything she needs to hear?" she asked.

"You are enough," I said. These were the words that came to mind after speaking with my mother. The perfectionist part of me wanted to be enough. I wanted to please my mother. That energy was controlling my throat space still.

"That's beautiful," Kate responded.

She walked me through the process of sending this energy to my mother, with this message wrapped in love and compassion.

"It was complex in there," Kate said, "but you are free of that now. If you need to do it again, you can." She paused to clear her throat.

"There is an intense cord attached there. It feels hot. Do you have some water that you can drink?" Kate asked.

I reached for my mason jar of water next to me.

"As you drink the water imagine it going down to the sacral space. It's a nice cooling element," I heard her breathing out heavily, clearing her throat space of energetic residue.

"There was some intense stuff going on," Kate said. "This is a process of creating sacred space for leaning into this and healing this thing. Your throat stuff is a big part of that. It's the big Kahuna."

I had to separate myself from judgment. I knew I was doing what I was meant to do. If I was disapproved of by others, that was separate from me. I needed to find my own support system that I yearned for.

I wiped the tears from my eyes.

"You may feel tired and emotions may come up. That's all normal. It may happen over the next couple of days. For some people it hits them later when it all settles in. Allow yourself to feel. You may need to cry. You may be angry. You may need to write something out," Kate said.

"Ok."

"Nurture yourself," she suggested. "Talk to your inner child. Look at how far you've come. Let her know that you're the adult now and are there to take care and support her."

The day following my call with Kate I felt exhausted, completely wiped out. I could barely move. I was taken back, yet again, about the power of energy work and how it could impact my physical body.

The cord cutting experience was intense. I'd released an energetic hold, and let go of fear, coming away with a clear visual that my soul wanted to escape my body.

I did what I could to come back down into it. The ground was unusually warm for February, so I took the opportunity to put my bare feet in the grass and soak up the sun.

I recalled Kate's reminder that the experience you have in your body is a gift. It's the way that your soul experiences this life, and there's always lessons to be learned.

Not long after my conversation with Kate, I released the *Peace with Endo Podcast* out into the world. I was finally ready for my voice to be heard.

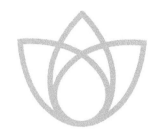

17. Roots

"In being true to yourself you will feel more alive, but you may also feel uncomfortable. This is because you are risking change! As you undergo certain changes, you may experience various intense emotions, such as fear, grief, or anger. Allow these emotions expression; after all, your inner guidance has to move through years of accumulated unconsciousness, denial, doubt, and fear. So let your feelings come up and wash through you—you are being cleared out and healed."

~ Shakti Gawain, Living in the Light

$\int$pring came again, and the cycle of rebirth showed in the world around me. As the year progressed, I paused to recognize that I'd had six subsequent starts to my period with only mild pain, as I'd imagined a "normal" period would be. This was a huge relief. Something had definitely shifted since getting deeper into the energy work. I'd experience a great amount of progress in a short time. Without those traumatic starts to my period, endometriosis felt more manageable. It wasn't as much of a disruption in my life.

I continued with the fresh organic celery juice in the morning. My digestion was stronger, my skin was glowing, and I had more energy than ever! I started to experiment with foods I had kept away from for many years, and found that they didn't bother me like they used to. It felt freeing to be able to eat what I wanted to sometimes, without worry.

Since starting my blog, each year I wrote about my experience with infertility for RESOLVE's national infertility awareness week® (NIAW), which happens in the last week of April. As the time rolled around again, I didn't even think about it. I didn't have much to say. I felt like a lot of the grief I'd experienced after years of struggle had released. My heart space felt better, like a weight had been lifted.

I found myself able to be truly happy for other women in my life who were having children. Looking at a newborn child, I could smile at its pure innocence and beauty, without feeling that horrible ache in my heart.

Finally, I was healing.

As the days continued to pass, and no child graced our lives, I took a step closer to accepting the idea that it wasn't going to happen. This was the end of the line. Maybe the female line ended with me, the sensitive one, with the power of my uterus spread out all over my body. It was time for me to feel it all. My soul was ready for Nirvana.

When I reasoned with myself, I saw the damage present in my body physically, emotionally, and energetically. It was too much for new life. What kind of pain would I be passing down? Was that selfish on my part?

I'd cracked the surface of what was going on at a deeper level, but I knew there was still much healing that needed to happen with my body, mind, and spirit.

In the meantime, I recognized that there was little sense fighting reality and stressing out about what I didn't have. I surrendered to the path that been placed in front of me. It seemed a different option was in store, one that I didn't expect, but one that could still be fulfilling in other ways. I learned to appreciate life as it was in the moment, and set my sights on other things.

I received a special invitation from Kate to join her new Open Soul™ Mastermind group. The program focused on chakra energy, how to work with it, and how to deepen your intuition. She taught how to tune into the energy field and the information it contained, so that I could be a healing guide for myself and others.

The program was based on the experiences that she had working with other people, along with her personal psychic knowledge and insight on a journey into the unseen territory of reality. She provided tools and meditations to access layers of soul energy that are always present under the surface, and right within reach.

Considering the huge role that she had on my healing journey, I was excited and ready to learn from Kate. I knew if I could help other endo sisters as much as she had helped me over the past six months, I'd be doing the world a great service. I was fascinated by her ability to see deeper into the souls of her clients, and I was ready to learn and explore how to do that.

There were three other women doing the program with me. I could relate to the stories of these women right away and could see that there was a reason why we'd been pulled together under Kate's wing.

In the first week of the program, Kate provided meditations to guide me in protecting my energy. Living as an empath all these years, this information was extremely valuable. I began to incorporate a protective visualization exercise every morning, before I interacted with clients over the phone, or before I went to public gatherings where the energy was often overwhelming. It didn't take long for me to see the benefits of this protection practice. It helped to keep me from picking up the energy of other people, and on a subconscious level, it helped me to feel safe.

The second session we had together in the mastermind was intense. It was emotional for me and it opened my eyes to just how much I feel things. As I'd explored this "feeling factor" throughout my life, I knew it was something I wasn't always open to. My patterns had led me to numb certain feelings. I understood I had to feel to heal, but that could get difficult when I felt so deeply.

I was reminded of this as I witnessed healing work Kate did with another woman in the group. As I tuned in and followed along, I could feel the pain of this woman deep in my heart space. This was accentuated because the pain was relatable to me. It was reflected to me.

I believe we are shown certain things in our life through

relationships and connections with other people that we need to see ourselves. I wasn't aware of this mirroring effect until I became a wellness coach and worked one-on-one with other endo sisters. I listened to their stories, their histories, and held space for the pain. As a result, I saw reflections of lessons I needed to see and feel, to help my own life situations. Sometimes it's harder to observe your own life when you're living within it. These women showed me what I needed to know.

Being in the new intimate group setting with Kate and these three other women, I could already see the mirroring effect happening. I related to all the women in different ways. After Kate had finished her session with this woman, I had an intense emotional release. I was sobbing, and I felt an ache in my heart as it all came out, like it was coming through me.

An empath feels other's pain and emotions as if they were their own, and it's a natural instinct to want to take that pain away, so we feel better. I was always wanting to help. What could I do to heal your pain? I felt the pain deeply within the endo community that I'd been an active member in for years, and I was called to help with it.

Kate helped me to see that I could use my empathic abilities and my compassionate pull to help to mirror the pain of my clients, to help them identify what's going on, and to help them release that.

After we learned how to protect ourselves, Kate moved us into exploring the root chakra. In an energetic sense the root chakra is the start of you, providing the foundation on which you build your life. It relates to ideas of stability, security, and your basic needs. When this chakra is open, you feel safe and fearless. When it's blocked, it throws everything off.

The place where the root chakra influenced my body at my

lower back and sacrum hurt... badly. I've had back issues for a long time, and I felt like it tied in with the pain in my pelvic region. I thought the chronic lower back pain stemmed from a trip to Oahu with Ryan, nearly a decade ago. I went back to the memory of that time, and pulled in the energetic statement that ached in my lower back.

Before we had flown out to Oahu, I missed taking a few days of birth control pills, and during that time I had sex with Ryan. I freaked out, convinced I was pregnant. I knew little about my body then. Somewhere along the line I'd missed the part about timing of ovulation and the science of how one actually got pregnant. All I knew was I'd had sex and missed a couple of pills.

That fear drove me to purchase a morning after pill. Looking back on that time, I saw how naive I was. I was completely disconnected from my body. Who knew what was in that pill? I regretted the decision as soon as the pill dropped into my throat. My fear drove it. My fear made me take that pill.

At the time I had little idea of how the morning after pill worked. I had the common misconception that it works like an abortion pill, and that I was killing new life. In reality it was a larger dose of the hormones I'd taken for years in the birth control pill. The morning after pill works by stopping implantation. It stops things before they start.

But I didn't know that. I thought I was putting in a pill that would kill the new life inside of me. My misguided decision was driven by fear. I was afraid of having a child. I wasn't ready. How would we ever make it with a kid? We weren't married. What would everyone think? Would that force us to get married? I wasn't ready for that.

The day after popping the pill, Ryan and I got on a plane to Oahu with his family. It was my first time there. We went to the beach, and I started to get really nauseated. When I got up, I lost my balance. I excused myself to the restroom and tried to make sense of the beautiful environment around me, which was being disrupted by sickness, of my own doing.

After resting for a bit on the beach, I started to feel better, so I joined Ryan in the ocean. It was March, the waves on the North Shore of the island were rough. I felt better jumping into them, feeling the salt on my skin and the sand in my toes. The force of the waves was strong. It didn't take long for me to get hit hard. I fell down, overcome by the wave, and my tailbone struck the floor of the ocean at full force. Bam. Ryan's strong arms pulled me out of the water, and he helped me back to solid ground.

My back and tailbone were super sore after the fall. After I returned home, I pulled something in my lower back lifting weights, which triggered the worst pain I'd felt in my life. My spine spasmed with shocks that kept me from moving an inch. I loaded up on pain pills and muscle relaxers, and tried not to move.

That pattern of back spasms and pain continued every couple of months. Eventually, my discomfort led to an MRI which showed two herniated discs in my lower back, one of which was hitting my sciatic nerve, causing the pain to cascade all the way down my legs and feet.

Surgery was suggested, but I decided not to go that route. I'd watched as a couple of co-workers had multiple back surgeries that only made things worse. That fed into my fear; I didn't want things to get worse.

The pain in my lower back prompted me to start doing yoga. I heard that it could help, and it did. The practice slowed me down, and put me in connection with my body and breath.

When I damaged my body in the ocean, my life changed. The water knocked me off my feet, and broke my root. I was met with the worst pain in my life, but it changed my trajectory. In seeking relief for my injury, I was introduced to the first path stone on a new journey to self-discovery, and the power of my breath.

While I could lessen the pain with yoga, it didn't go away. The ache was a reminder of that day in the water and the decision I'd made the day before, driven by a deeply rooted fear.

Kate introduced us to her root chakra meditation, which included a visualization exercise that looked deeper at the primary parts of that energy center, which include safety and security, your home, body, and money. The root also deals with your tribe, which covers your family of origin, your upbringing, and those who are around you now. The visualization walked through each of these roots to see how they look. Are they sturdy? Was there anything wrong with them?

Only days before I first listened to Kate's root meditation, there was a series of powerful rain storms that knocked off one of the downspouts on our house located above the window well for the basement. As a result, a downpour of flash flood rain dropped right around the house.

On the morning following one of the storms, I woke up, went down into the basement, and felt water under my feet. The carpet was soaked. My mind went to the worst. I had visions of my home's foundation cracking in front of my eyes, with water coming through those cracks.

Ryan spent a majority of his life in the basement. That's where his man cave was. The flooding disrupted our home environment, and came with added uncertainty, and the stress of fixing our old home. Foundation issues were a big deal. How would we afford that? It felt like it was all crumbling in front of me.

What could be done now to solve the situation? My rational mind thought. The water had shown up in the basement after the fallen downspout. If we fixed it, that should solve the problem for the moment, and it wouldn't hurt to check the rest of the gutters.

That morning was stressful. After I discovered the water intrusion, woke Ryan, and endured the disruption that followed, I picked a card from my oracle deck and spoke aloud the question that I usually asked,

"What do I need to know today?"

The card that popped up was "Purification". It was an image of a woman who held a dove in one of her hands, a symbol of peace, as she stood in waves of water. Purification. Was that what was happening?

My vision of the cracked and leaking foundation was the mirroring impact of my messed-up root, in full effect.

I found a gutter company recommended by someone in my neighborhood, and they came out the next day to give me a quote. The day they were scheduled to come back, it snowed. It was a heavy spring snow, heavy and wet, covering the trees and budding flowers with a blanket of white. I assumed the gutter company wasn't going to come out to do the work that day, but I didn't hear from them. A part of me was glad they didn't show up, because I wanted to call around and get some other quotes before they came back. I figured they would call to re-schedule a time.

The following evening, I went through Kate's root chakra meditation. I took a look at my roots in each of the areas: safety and security, my body, home, and money. When I got to the safety and security root, I noticed it was smooth, and nearly transparent. I reached for it, but I couldn't hold on.

I fell back into the darkness. I literally felt it happen.

The next day I settled at my desk for the start of a new workweek. I was getting ready to get on a work call when I heard my dogs going crazy up in the front room. I knew the sound of their barks indicated that someone was at the house.

I peeked through the lower level window to see who was there, and spotted the work truck for the gutter company I'd called the week before, the ones that hadn't shown up or called when the snow came through. Here they were, unannounced. I heard the doorbell ring, but I didn't answer it. I wasn't happy with the fact that they'd blown me off, and I wasn't sure that I wanted them to do the work anymore. I intended to call around and get more quotes. Plus, I had a work call I needed to take.

I figured when I didn't answer the door, they would go away, but the opposite happened. I watched one of the workers disappear to the side of the house, where the gate was to the backyard. *It's locked, he's not going to be able to get back there,* I thought. Why would he? He wasn't invited. I let the women who did the quote for us know they needed to call us first before showing up. We had dogs that had free access to the yard, and I wasn't sure what would happen when a stranger came to the fence.

The locked gate was not enough to deter the men. A moment later I watched as they leaned a ladder up against the house and got up on the roof. That action triggered me. What did they think they were doing? I had not authorized them to be there! I picked up my cell phone and dialed the office to the company. When the woman answered my mouth exploded with anger.

"Is this how you conduct business?" I yelled. I was flabbergasted at their lack of professionalism.

"Get them the fuck off my roof!" I screamed. My entire body was shaking. My home had been violated. Yet another factor of my root space.

A couple hours after my intense outburst I got on a call with Kate and the other ladies in the mastermind group. Kate walked us through the root exercise again. My lower back was aching. As I did the exercise a lot of emotions came up. I was sobbing. It was the water coming up again, breaking through.

I told them about the reaction I'd had with the men on my roof, and how out of character it was for me to freak out like that. I was angry. I felt violated. My home was supposed to be a haven for safety. What gave them the right to do that?

"It was like they raped us," Ryan said later.

His words reflected what I was thinking, which brought back the immensity of the energetic imprint rape had on my system, and it pissed me off. I think that anger needed to be felt, and released.

All of this transpired while I was exploring my root chakra. Plenty came up — factors of safety, security, money, and the connection with my body. Your body's what's grounded to the earth, it's what's rooted here, but when you live in a body that brings pain that's not always easy.

I thought back to the visualization Kate had given me months before, with the image of my soul flying above my body like a parachute, with these stakes into the ground, holding on... barely... as if my soul was trying to escape my body. That hit home for me, living with endo, within a body that can bring pain, and wanting to escape it.

After the group call with Kate ended, I came away with revelations of the root, of it cracking through. What happens when the root breaks the ground? It grows into a plant, or into a flower. It starts with a seed. It starts with you. It starts with the roots, but it has to eventually break that plane. It has to come up and break through the earth to become a living being. It has to flourish.

I was reminded, yet again, of the power of energy work, of mirroring what I needed to learn, feel, and release.

Following that intense group session and emotional release with exploration of my root, I had a call with one of my one-on-one clients. She brought up the same issue: pain in her lower back, with her root. I kid you not. It was the same pain presented to me, in unison, as all of this was going on bringing attention to these things.

I received the message loud and clear! I was aware that my root was messed, up and that things needed to release so that the roots could break through, grow, blossom, and flourish into something beautiful... from darkness to light.

18. Shadow

"No tree, it is said, can grow to heaven unless
its root reach down to hell."

~ Carl Jung

$\mathcal{D}$uring the first time I did Kate's root chakra visualization meditation, I took a look at my security root and it was thin and shiny. I reached for it, but it slipped right through my hands. I had a distinct feeling of falling backwards into the darkness.

The darkness didn't leave. It lingered long after the day I freaked out on the gutter guys, and broke down in hysterical tears at the end of Kate's mastermind call. Thoughts came into my head I hadn't had in a long time, dark ones, resounding around the narrative... *I don't matter, none of this matters.*

I knew in my conscious mind that wasn't true, but I couldn't shake the thought. I cried a lot of tears and felt this horrible ache in my heart space. I think it was triggered by exploring my root chakra, where my soul's existence took shape into human form.

There's a lot that can come up in that space. Psychologist Carl Jung related the root chakra to what he called the collective unconsciousness, which encompasses past energies, going deeper into your ancestry. Looking into the dark parts, he said, will eventually help you find the light.

Jung said that the Self cannot be healed and whole unless we look at and acknowledge the "shadow"; the part that we are unwilling to look into, that which has been buried within us all. That includes everything you dislike about yourself.

Everyone has these fears. You hold them deep in your subconscious. It could be feelings that you're unlovable, unworthy, or broken. The desire for approval runs deep. We identify with the opinions of others, especially authority figures whose opinions you can hear as your own.

It takes a lot of energy to continue keeping the shadow buried, and to suppress the multitude of fears. The result of that energy is depletion. The more fear you hold onto, the more fearful situations are attracted into your life.

When it's looked at and acknowledged, the shadow no longer has power, no longer unconsciously runs you. Once you become acquainted with the shadow, you no longer have to project your fears on the world. You lose interest in crime, violence, and fearful disasters. When you turn attention from the screen, inward to your mind, then attraction from such things disappears.

I'd definitely pierced the shadow deep in my root space. It was overwhelming. *None of this matters.* I retreated from social media and my other modes of expression to the Peace with Endo community. I had thoughts of deleting my existence on the Internet. I wanted to disappear.

The next morning, I woke up to a memory, or perhaps a message. It popped into my head... *The Forgotten.* The thought made my eyes widen.

Shortly before Jeff died, we went to see a movie at the theaters: *The Forgotten.* The film is about a mother whose son disappears. It's as if he never existed. No one around remembered him. A strange feeling lingered with me after watching that film, and then being witness to the death of a man I loved. One day he was here, the next he was gone.

I wasn't sure why the memory came to mind. I hadn't thought about that movie in years, but it made me feel sick. *The Forgotten.*

In the days to come I cried a lot of tears, enough to give myself a near permanent headache and puffy eyes. I couldn't explain the deep amount of grief that was releasing from me. It was intense, deep, darkness.

Perhaps you've been in that space, too. It was during this time when I heard the news of another suicide in the endo community. It wasn't someone I knew personally, but I saw that she was local to my area. My heart ached in understanding.

I pulled back from doing anything with my business, or any creative endeavors. I crumpled up my to-do lists, and directed my attention towards reading. I let my mind travel to fantasylands, taking over the drama of someone else's story. Over the course of two weeks, I devoured eight books.

I mentioned my discontentment to Kate and the other ladies in the mastermind group that I felt lost about my direction and purpose in this life. I shared my thoughts of deleting my existence on the Internet. Maybe it was time to start something new? The thought continued to eat at the back of my mind. *None of this matters.*

Kate walked me through a visualization exercise where I was in a white room and there were three choices in front of me. Which had the most pull? I came to a blank. I couldn't see what I wanted to do. I felt totally lost.

She and the other women in the group confirmed what I was not able to see. The choice my soul energy was drawn to was the writing. I needed to write this book.

I scoffed at the thought. "Writing isn't going to allow me to quit my day job," I said. It felt like a waste of time. Frustration kicked in.

"You never know," Kate said.

I started my period a couple of days later. The pain I felt in the tub that day was more emotional than physical. It stirred up the question: Why? It didn't feel like anything mattered. I was ready to disappear to another dimension as the kid did in *The Forgotten*.

Life with endometriosis made me no stranger to suffering. It was what led me to further spiritual exploration that connected me to the core message of The Buddha — life is suffering. Through the teachings of the Buddha, and many other spiritual mentors to follow, I learned mindfulness and living in the present moment. That, after all, was the way to combat feelings of anxiety and depression which were generally rooted in thoughts of the past, or of the future.

But what if the now sucks? As I soaked in the tub that day, it did. I couldn't get over the darkness that had come over my mind.

I brought a new book along with me to read in the warm water. It was called *Man's Search for Meaning* by Viktor Frankl. The book shared Frankl's experiences as an Auschwitz concentration camp inmate during World War II.

Talk about suffering.

Frankl explained how he was able to survive the horrible living conditions and brutal work he had to complete each day as a prisoner. He described the differences between the inmates who made it out, and those who died inside, sheer luck notwithstanding.

The difference came from purpose. Those that made it through were able to initiate forward thinking, beyond their existing circumstances. They took hold of something they felt positively about, and then imagined the outcome.

For Frankl, his purpose came from a manuscript he was working on before he was taken to the camps. He had it with him, his most prized possession, but it was taken from him along the way. Completing the book gave him a reason to keep going.

An even stronger pull from the inmates who survived came from love. They had someone on the outside that they dreamed about seeing again. They imagined themselves having a nice meal together, or sleeping together in a warm bed. The visualization of finding that peaceful place again, carried them through their now, which was full of suffering and misery.

Love is what matters. Hold onto that.

Reading Frankl's story got me thinking more about my own purpose, and the book I'd been writing for the past couple of years. The book had been pulling at me to release it, but my energy had been scattered. I was trying to do too many things.

I directed my energy back towards creation, and made a commitment to myself to get a draft of the book down. I wrote for hours every day, spilling out my soul into paragraphs and pages of prose. My attention became laser focused.

After only a few days of writing, I started to feel much better. Writing helped me to process everything that had happened, and to release all that was coming to the surface. I started to see the greater lessons to be learned in this life, and how endometriosis has been one of my greatest teachers.

Writing helped me to heal on a much deeper level. The words brought my soul into a physical existence. It was my way of expressing what needed to flow out of me, bringing the energy of my thoughts into physical existence. It served as a gateway to my inner being.

There was a moment during this time when I felt the darkness lift. I sat out in the backyard, in my spot in the sun, and a little white feather dropped to my feet. I take feathers as a sign from the angels, and a reminder that I'm safe and protected now. Everything's going to be okay.

My two-week retreat from my social media and blogging gave me space to return back to me. When I started to write again it was with purpose. That spark re-lit my life and helped dispel the darkness. I'd pulled back into the energy of creation in the divine feminine, allowing the words to flow through me, releasing stagnation, and raising my vibe. I was back in alignment with what I was here to do. Write. Create. Be.

As the book poured out of me, I put the pieces of the puzzle together, taking a bigger look at the past year of my life, and seeing how I had completely transformed. I felt like a caterpillar that had finally broken free into the beauty of the butterfly. In fact, I saw an orange butterfly consistently over this time, flying in and out of my vision as I spent days outside, soaking up the summer sun.

Kate mentioned butterflies and dragonflies multiple times during readings she did on me during the group program. Both are signs of transformation. It was clear to me after coming out of the darkness that I needed to address the shadow in order to see the light.

19. Soul Lessons

"Remembering the past-life trauma or event that has resulted in a current-life physical symptom is often enough the cure."

~ Dr. Brain Weiss, Miracles Happen:
The Transformational Healing Power of Past-Life Memories.

*A*fter turning that big corner, I had another group call in the mastermind group with Kate and the other ladies. She let us know beforehand the main purpose of the call was to practice tuning into each other's energy.

I was still new at doing so, though I could definitely sense other people's energy in my body. I learned to tune into my empathic abilities, and related the physical sensations I felt with the different chakra areas. I also started to have some vague images come through.

I practiced tuning into my own energy the night before the call. I sat outside under the summer evening sky, closed my eyes, then grounded and protected my energy with an opening blessing. I imagined my roots going deep into the earth, and protected myself with a white light that went around my whole body like a shield. Once that was in place, I lit a fire around that shield.

I took a deep breath into my heart space and relaxed my body. Then, I shifted my breath and attention to flow up my chakras toward my third eye space. Within this field of inner vision, I saw an image of a tower.

On our group call the next day, I was happy to report that I was doing much better and making great progress on my book. I'd dedicated a couple of hours each day to writing. It was my main focus. Everything else was on hold.

As we moved into the energy reading part of the call, Kate asked me what I wanted to know, "It's helpful if we have a clear question to focus on. The more specific the reading can be."

I had to think about it. After experiencing major emotional release in our calls the past few weeks, I was feeling good. I was in sync with my writing. I felt purposeful.

"Is there anything that I haven't written yet that should be included in my book?" I asked.

Silence followed as everyone tuned into my energy. What did it have to say? When I felt into myself, I noticed an ache at my solar plexus region right away. Personal power. I made note of the sensation, a reminder that this was a primary message I wanted to get across to you.

I listened to the ladies give me excellent guidance on what to include and how to handle my energy as I moved closer to birthing this book into the world.

Kate was the last to report what she saw and felt. I didn't expect what came next.

"I saw a past life or two. In one you were locked in a tower. In another you were down in a well. So, it's like tower in the air, tower in the earth, making you dive both ways," she said.

The tower. I got the same image the night before.

"You're locked away in punishment in the first one, for not giving someone something that they want. The other one you drowned in this place and all this icky stuff was around and it's come into this life with you and it comes out your throat. It's murky, like what you would have felt with that coming into your lungs."

Kate felt the experience of this in her body.

"I'm so uncomfortable. Solar plexus. You had your power taken away," she said.

I nodded in recognition. The same message had come through my body. I felt the ache there.

"Inhale into your solar plexus. Bring that air into your chest and out your throat," she exhaled out loud through her mouth.

"I'm watching this muck leaving me. I didn't want to clear it without you knowing," Kate said.

My pain was impacting her because she wanted to make me aware of it. I was grateful for that, but not that she'd picked up the muck from me.

Kate implored, "I want you to inhale air, not water, into your throat. Let the water come out of your lungs, 'ahhhh' and the sludge."

I followed along, trying to release the energy from my throat space. My throat was super sore. It wasn't like that before.

"Can you hum? Your voice was not heard," she said.

There was power in those words. My voice hadn't been heard. That played out in this life, too.

"You've had multiple throat wounds."

My hands went to my throat, which had been a source of trouble for as long as I could remember — sore throats, swollen tonsils and glands. I was diagnosed with Hashimoto's, and a nodule on the right side of my thyroid.

Kate continued, "I need to re-center myself. That was unexpected to see a past life or two. Breathe in through the top of the head, exhale it all the way down, feel it flow into every cell of your being. Let it wind down your spine. Bring the earth energy back up. Then exhale out the top of your head. Inhale into your heart space. Wonderful."

I drowned in a well. I couldn't crawl out. The thought lingered in my head, sending shivers through my body. It sounded like something from a horror movie.

"It's not good. It's heavy," Kate confirmed. "It's part of the reason why there's a physical ailment down in your lower chakras. I've wanted to know this. It's not just this life stuff. It's a manifestation from a past life. I was not expecting that. It's very emotional."

I felt it too, heavy in my heart space. I'd said something someone didn't like and was punished for it, multiple times.

Kate walked me through a clearing exercise to help remove the muck from both her and me. My throat was throbbing all the way into my ears. I had a memory stuck there. Kate described them as tiny threads that attached from my throat up to my ears, and through the drainage tubes of my ears and lymph nodes. That came from breathing in muck from the water.

The water. The space where I'd had many a spiritual experience, a place in which I'd felt like I was ready to die. The shallow water in the tub was the place where I died while still alive.

"You have not released these memories from your past life, hanging on like a thread. It's very tight," Kate said.

I could sense her discomfort, as she felt my pain.

"You are not 100% but we've done all that your body can handle for now," she told me.

I came away with a loud reminder that my soul was ready to be heard. I needed to find my voice, and revive my personal power. It was the same message I too had received over the past six months. Kate brought it to light, and gave a much deeper meaning to it all.

After the call was over, I experienced many emotions. Past life experience? While I'd considered the notion, I wasn't sure if it was true. It was beyond what I'd learned as a child about heaven and hell. Reincarnation?

I was always drawn to Eastern philosophies. The reincarnation idea came up in my studies of the teachings from the Buddha. It came from the notion that we all have a lesson to learn in our time here on earth. The ultimate goal of Nirvana came with a true awakening of spirit to enlightenment, where suffering finally goes away. There is peace, and the re-birth process stops. Peace prevails.

Another theory is that we hold inherited memories. Modern science has only decoded a very small portion of our genetic code. It's thought that these memories can live somewhere along this strand. Cellular memories and traits are passed down from previous generations that may not necessarily be within your bloodline. As your eye color and other natural instincts are coded here, so too are inherent beliefs and tendencies.

Your genetic code is not fixed. It can be modified. Your body and mind are influenced by hereditary illnesses, cultural behavior patterns, inherited religious dogmas or fears, past traumas, major life events, disasters, and other environmental factors.

The idea is similar, in a way, to what I'd found in Mark Wolynn's book, *It Didn't Start with You*. Kate pulled up energy that was living in my energetic field, be that from a past life, or inherited memories. It shook me up, because I related to it.

She handed me a big soul lesson. My throat energy was wounded. I'd lost my power and my voice. It was drowned out. I felt the grief and loss in my heart space as the right side of my throat throbbed.

I didn't know what to do with myself that night, as I paced the room trying to process all the emotions that were coming through me. I went outside to the backyard and soaked up the remnants of the evening sun. It was the same spot, a night before, where I'd seen a vision of a tower. Kate confirmed it with her reading on me. She also mentioned multiple sightings of the dragon, my spirit guide and a powerful protective being that shot fire.

Something triggered in my long-term memory... *The Eyes of the*

Dragon. I recalled my mother reading this book to my brothers and me as a child. Something about the story had sparked my attention. The dragon?

I rose up and went inside to search for the old book. I pulled its tattered cover from the shelf, brushing off a layer of dust. It'd been a long time since I'd last opened it. I'd written my name on the outside spine when I was a girl, 'AUBREE' with a little heart next to it.

I brought the book back outside with me and started to read. As I progressed into the story, I came across little bookmarks I'd stuck in the pages years before. One was a game piece from a fast-food restaurant. I flipped it over and noticed the expiration date at the bottom: 1998. I was 16. I was about to get mono from my boyfriend, which would permanently change my throat space, and I was on the cusp of a large disruption in my personal power when I lost my virginity to an evil man. *That's ironic*, I thought.

I devoured the story from my childhood that encompassed messages of good and evil, the balance between light and shadow. The villain was a dark magician who was advisor to the King. The King had two sons, Peter and Thomas. The younger, Thomas, was conceived through a rough sexual encounter. I'll say it for what it was — rape.

The magician didn't get along with Peter, who was heir to the throne, so he took evil measures to frame him for the murder of his father. Peter was found guilty and as punishment, was sent to the top of a tower.

The tower.

My throat was still throbbing the next day, enough for me to reach out to Kate. Her throat was still sore, too. She suggested tending to the physical part that was sore by drinking herbal tea with lemon and honey. She reminded me that there was a lot of emotion that needed to be released from my heart space, too.

Kate messaged me, *"I believe that a part of you is still remembering this past life experience of dying and not knowing how to move on from life to the afterlife. It was a bit of a denial and major confusion. Not realizing you were out of body."*

Her words made the visual of my lost soul come to mind. *The Forgotten.* The memory made my heart ache. The intense emotions that came up when I first explored my root space came together. I literally felt myself fall back in the darkness, as one would feel being dropped into the well, drowning, lost at the bottom of the earth.

My energy levels were extremely low. The fatigue kept me from doing much but think about the revelations Kate had given to me. My throat continued to ache throughout that day, and into the night. I couldn't focus on much of anything. A lot of emotions came out. Water poured down my cheeks.

The scars of past lives were manifesting into my existence here. The past pain was finally acknowledged, and it pieced together so much. I wasn't heard, my power was taken away; I was no stranger to these lessons.

As I looked back on my life, I saw how this suppression and loss of personal power had played out in my life. It showed up in a big way when I expressed my spiritual truth to my father before I married Ryan. That instance was terrifying at the time, but it started me on a path of personal discovery to figure out who I was, and what I believed in.

That was followed by a diagnosis of endometriosis — a condition I'd never heard of. How? I struggled with excruciating pain with my periods from the start, and was told over and over again that it was normal, that it was part of being a woman. I didn't talk about it. Since pain was all I knew, it became my normal.

I mentioned the pain frequently to my gynecologists over the years, but it was written off, dismissed as a common discomfort of womanhood. There's a subconscious impact that comes from not feeling like you're heard, feeling like your voice doesn't matter.

None of this matters, I don't matter. I remembered the dark thoughts that I knew weren't the true me, but it was hard to shake them. I think I rattled them up from my subconscious mind, from this expansive unknown part of the brain where soul energy intermingles with ancestral energy and past trauma.

It felt as if that root energy cracked open. It'd happened in mirroring effect right before my eyes as water came up through the foundation of my home, which was later violated by uninvited guests. That triggered a lot of anger. I didn't understand all the emotions at the time. I was being shown these same lessons in real time. Synchronicity.

Water is the element of the sacral space, which is directly connected to the throat chakra. The two are influenced physically by the vagus nerve, and vibration between the two came through in sound. It was time to find my truth.

Kate followed up with me the next day to make sure I was okay. My throat was still sore.

"I had to sing today. I have a song for you that will mend your throat. I was told to send it to you for healing. It worked for me today. Hum along with it even if you aren't sure of the words. Once you have them memorized sing louder and feel it in your body like a strong Ohm sound, except it's the sound of the song. It will release things. You will feel it go. Relief," Kate said.

I followed her suggestions. With my headphones on, and the sound strongly vibrating in my throat, I learned the words to the song. I sang them out, *"See the sun..."*

"What are you doing?" Ryan asked, hearing my hums through the floor. "A new type of meditation?"

"Kate told me to sing this song to heal my throat," I said, with a giggle. I could tell from the rise of his eyebrows that I need say no more. I shared some of this stuff with Ryan, but most of it I processed on my own. He wasn't as receptive to the energy work as I was. It took some convincing.

The song worked. My throat energy opened up, and the tightness released.

My throat started to hurt again a couple of weeks later. I woke up from a dream in which I received a gift from a mystical being, and when I opened the box it was a bright blue shining light, the color of the throat chakra space. Then I woke up.

Later that day, I had an encounter with a red robin. While I was sitting outside, it landed a few feet away, and stared right at me. My dogs kept chasing it out of the yard, but it returned three or four times. I went inside to look up the robin in my *Pocket Guide to Spirit Animals* book and there was a line about, "singing your song."

When I went back outside, the red robin was there again! It sat on the edge of the tree branch, and again was looking directly at me. So, I sang a song to it. It seemed to like that.

The next day during meditation, I saw a vision of a frog. I looked up to see what that meant, and there was a line saying that singing or chanting will help you feel better. I received an obvious message; use your voice. Sing. Open up that throat chakra space. Express yourself.

Looking back, I see that this lesson was presented to me as a young girl on Saturday nights at church As I listened to my mother's voice ring through the sanctuary, connecting her soul with the glory of God. Her voice was beautiful, and showed me the way early on: choir, singing, harmony. It made me feel alive. Turns out it was necessary. I needed to clear all the gunk from my heart space and find my voice, the sound of my soul.

I finished up my nostalgic reading of *The Eyes of the Dragon*, blown away by the symbols that'd shown up in the story, as they played out in the longer story of my soul. Peter was locked in the tower by the evil magician. His voice was silenced.

Spoiler alert: Peter makes it out of the tower, with help from a lot of patience, as he builds a long rope from threads of the napkins he gets at his meals. The tower is high in the sky, so he needs a very long rope. It takes him a long time to collect enough thread to intertwine it together — thin, yet strong.

I thought back to the threads in my throat space, and the vision Kate gave me of being locked in a tower, confirmed by my own intuitive vision of a tower in the sky. My other past life showed death from water, deep in the earth. I'd been silenced in both ends.

The thin thread doesn't hold Peter all the way down the tower. It breaks, and he falls backwards. Luckily his friends are there to support his fall. I saw the symbolism in my own story. My roots were shaky. It was obvious I needed further support.

My curiosity about past life regression led me to Dr. Brian Weiss, a psychotherapist who was astonished and skeptical when one of his patients started to recall past-life traumas that seemed to hold the key to her recurring nightmares and anxiety attacks. She began to channel messages from "the spaces between lives", which contained remarkable revelations about Dr. Weiss' family and his dead son. Using past-life regression therapy, he was able to heal the patient.

I saw that he'd written many books on past life regressions. I picked one up called *Miracles Happen: The Transformational Healing Power of Past-Life Memories.* The book was full of other people's past life recollections in connection with Dr. Weiss. The many stories and perspectives helped to shift my own way of thinking, with recognition that there are deeper soul lessons to be learned in this life on earth. Once these lessons are acknowledged, it's amazing how, for many, physical pain drifts away. When you realize the energy, that information no longer has an unconscious effect; you can feel it, and let it go.

It was time to mend the past pain, which I came to believe was all connected within my heart space. The fourth chakra is at the middle of the seven energy centers, uniting the lower chakras of matter, and the upper chakras of spirit. The heart chakra is spatial, but it also serves as a bridge between your body, mind, emotions, and spirit. It's your source of love and connection. Within the heart space, your purpose comes forth. It's directly connected, energetically and physically, to your sacral space, the center of creation.

Why did a soul come back into a body that had a lot of pain? Why would my soul choose to live with endometriosis? I came away with a wise answer to these questions after reading *Miracles Happen.*

It was a lesson on receiving.

Endometriosis forced me to slow down, to take care of myself. I had no other choice.

Once I opened up to receive love, help, guidance, and

abundance, it all came to me. Once I verbally declared this intention, my energy shifted. Even when everything else was closed, my crown was still open. Synchronicity happened. New people came into my life. I was directed to energy workers and healers who made a huge difference in a short amount of time, and was directed to wise teachers whose words filled my heart chakra. I surrendered to the process, allowing myself to feel. I'd released blocks in my energy meridians causing things to flow again.

Opening up allowed space to let go. The emotional release was extreme, as if I was feeling all the pain from these experiences that I hadn't allowed myself to feel along the way. I physically felt the memories of past trauma that needed to be felt and acknowledged, so that they could finally leave me.

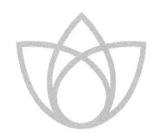

20. Echo

"Grief loves the hollow; all it wants is to hear its own echo."

~ Hisham Matar, In the Country of Men

The calendar switched to "eclipse season". A lunar eclipse was followed by a total solar/lunar eclipse that crossed coast-to-coast for the first time since 1918. All eclipses are about letting go, but the powerful total solar and lunar eclipse meant something significant was ready to be released.

The full eclipse cast a long shadow across the Earth's surface. Some say it was the universe's way of clearing energy that needed to come up. The shadow needs to be addressed if release is to happen, and as the sun and the moon crossed paths perfectly, it stood as a reminder of the power and connection between masculine and feminine energies: the sun and the moon, the fire and the water, the yin and the yang. There was a call for balance, and in order for that to happen, old stagnant energy needed to be cleared. It was the perfect time to do so.

I sat outside under the mid-day sky as the eclipse reached its peak. We weren't in the direct path of it, so I only received a taste of the shadow. I moved to my seat outside and meditated under the strange, slightly darkened sky. I opened my eyes from meditation shortly before the peak eclipse time, and took a long breath in. The buzz of insects surrounded me. The summer crickets sang their song. I could feel their vibration, the hum, a flapping of wings in unison.

A short time later, the sky went back to its bright blue, and the world moved on.

Later that day, I had a call with the mastermind group. There were only two ladies on that day: Kate and Bethan.

"I was meditating, and you popped into my awareness. I saw you singing," Kate said.

I nodded with a smile. The singing had helped, but my throat still felt murky and gross. As the call progressed, I found myself having to clear my throat often.

Kate asked us if we'd done the guided visualization meditation she provided called, Water of Truth. The focus was on the throat chakra, and the water connection with the sacral chakra.

"What came up for you?" Kate asked.

"The first time I did it I was at a water park flying down one of those tubes. At the end of it I dumped into a pool of water. The second time I did it I was at a lake, floating in a tube," I said.

"Interesting," Kate said. "How did that make you feel?"

I thought back to the feeling of flying down the water slide. I never much enjoyed the experience of all that water splashing up in my face, going down to an unknown space, holding my breath for the impact.

"Out of control," I said, clearing my throat again.

"My throat space feels murky. It's sticky, like there's something in there physically," I said.

"I can take a look around, see what's going on there. Do you have a specific question?" Kate asked.

"My ultimate question is what do I do? How do I break through the stuff in my throat?" I asked.

Kate closed her eyes and tuned into my energy.

I closed mine, too.

"You need to rest emotionally. Take time out from trying to explore all the stuff that's coming up and let one thing at a time. Too much at once. Continually slow down, even slower."

"Yeah," I agreed.

"If you were swimming across a lake and you got tired and started panicking you would drown. If you paused and relaxed and rested, you'd survive. You really have to wait. That's what's going on," Kate said. "I can feel the blockages in the throat space."

She took a breath in, "I'm checking your heart space to see if there's anything else here."

Silence followed as Kate explored.

"Interesting. Gratitude or worship towards knowing this information. I saw you down on your knees like you were praying."

"Knowing something specific? The truth?" I asked.

"Specifically?" Kate repeated. She paused.

"This is weird sounding. I saw you putting decayed leaves into your mouth. Whatever is clogged here, starting to take it out. It's a very heavy, gross feeling. Gross in the throat. A bear came up and stuck its snout in your face," she paused to look up the symbolism of the bear. "Set clear boundaries. Ask for what you want. Take some time out from your usual routine to spend in solitude. That makes sense to me. That's so fascinating."

"You're on a forest floor in the throat chakra space. There's a feeling of a continuous cycle, like a Ferris wheel. It looks like a constant cycle, but it's very slow. I think it could be time to get off of that," she said.

"I'm going into your third eye space. More struggle. There's a sense of not being able to get out of water. Climbing up a rope that's swaying around. It's not very stable in the third eye. I saw another animal that should be swimming, but it wasn't," she stopped to look up the symbolism of the animal.

"No matter what's happening in your life do whatever it takes to keep your faith strong. It's important right now to trust your life circumstances, and surrender to the will of spirit, trusting that it will all work out. You'll soon find clarity and purpose in this confusion that you're experiencing. Focus on the fact that life is a sacred gift and find ways to express your gratitude in as many ways as possible. Whatever changes you're going through, go with the flow. It was the swan just keeping its neck out of the water. It felt like it was not... safe.

"Lots of animals right now. The otter comes out as well. Time to relax, be more playful, spontaneous, creative. Whatever struggles you're facing now, face them head on with courage and tenacity.

"There's a layer of protection and debris over your throat space. We've already done some deep healing here. So, I'm not sure what else is coming up there, or if it's moving from another space. It's almost like an infection that's making its way out of the body. The throat would be the most logical space for it to be coming out of."

I took a long breath into my throat space.

Kate continued, "Let's see what else comes up here. It feels like a fish out of water... a big fish out of water."

The line went quiet as Kate dug deeper.

"I see around you is a situation where you're being dragged around against your will. Not having a say in this matter. I don't know if this is a past life energy that's coming in. It seems to be. There's a feeling of hands not being able to move. I don't know what happens after that..." Kate's voice cut off as she took a long breath.

"Do you have connections to any of your past life stuff?" she asked.

"No, but I find that all to be fascinating," I said. I told them about the book *Miracles Happen*, and all the stories of people who were able to heal from physical ailments by experiencing past life traumas.

"The biggest influence over this that could have manifested into this life is not having control over your body and losing your life in a violent way. This is a lot of people's story. It's giving me a really big headache because you've had your head hit a lot. So uncomfortable," Kate's voice dropped off.

"You've given me a visual before of being dragged," I said.

"Have I?" Kate asked.

Kate didn't remember most of the readings that she gave to people. It's like she went into another state of consciousness.

"You gave me a vision of my younger self being dragged by the head," I said.

"I think it's more than that. Definitely more than that. It's a man that's isolated in a forest. It's part of it for some reason. It creates a massive headache around my head. I'm uncomfortable with this space. I'm not sure if there's any more purpose in that, except to see how it's influencing your body," Kate said.

Kate asked if she could energetically be in my presence, and talked me through different hand positions and visualizations through my head space, guided with direction of my breath and awareness.

"Notice whatever you notice. Anything that seems wobbly or unstable, go ahead and stabilize it with your heart. Envision the energy around those spaces as if they're piecing back together fragments of your energy that's been spilling out, leaking out and reinforced by pain in this life. You've come into this world with this energetic drainage that you've come to put back together here," she said.

I allowed my breath to carry me through Kate's instructions and visualizations.

"This past life thing has carried with you. It's impacted all three of your upper chakras for your whole life. I see it's always been that way," Kate said.

She was right. I always had headaches as a child. I still do. My head is tender in many areas. Was that all discomfort manifested from old soul pain? The memories released in my energy.

"It echoes in this life," Kate continued. "You can release yourself from it, because all of your situations are not here anymore. It's not part of this life. Situations in your life have echoed it to make you feel it. A really loud echo. It's like you couldn't get closure in that life, right? So, you have a chance to do that now."

"What I've taken from all of this…" I paused to clear my throat, "…expression is a big part. Using my voice. Whether that be through music or speaking. I've been put in a group of women, the women that I'm speaking to at this moment have lost their voices. Being put in this situation, I don't have control over my body. Endo is mysterious and painful and related to sexuality. It's like a way to give a voice to these women that aren't being heard."

Kate took a deep breath, "I'm not ignoring you. I'm siphoning off the emotions that come with all of this. I feel the intense grief and suffering in this aspect. It's like a crosshair on your head. I'm sending it back to earth. It hits you right in the gut/sacral. That's to be expected with this sort of thing."

I watched as she cleared the energy from her body.

"Let's see what else is going on with that. Everything is buzzing. How are you feeling?"

"I feel pressure there," I said, bringing attention to the lower half of my body.

"I've got a song. You and the Tori Amos songs," she chuckled. "It's called *Horses*. You need to listen to that. It's a very cryptic song. I'm tearing up, but that's okay. Don't worry. Empath stuff." Kate sniffled, "It's a strong song in a way, but also tragic. It's like the theme song for this experience in a weird way. I see you getting on the horse, taking the power from this space. It's a good sign of a shift to power from discombobulation.

"You're still remembering the pain. It's a feeling of head hitting the ground. That doesn't feel good, ever. I don't know if you've ever hit your head or anything? It's the jarring feeling in the head and neck. It seems to come in the right side quite a bit. I'm feeling a lot of stuff on this side. Where are we going with this?" Kate stopped for a moment.

"The song will teach you about coming back to yourself, finding yourself and knowing that the person in the past that will find light in this life. There's a line that says, 'The threads that are golden don't break easily.' What should she do next?" she mumbled.

"To process today's stuff, get as naked as you feel you can, and get in a cozy blanket like a cocoon. You're safe. Allow your head space to show you what's going on. There's a lot of pain on that side physical from this past life experience."

"That's always where I have my pain. All the way down the right side of my body," I confirmed. My right side almost always ached.

"You need to cry. Like for her. I'm trying to let some of it out for you. It transmutes when I do this stuff," Kate said, as tears rolled down her cheeks.

"You know that feeling when you're so upset, and you can't breathe? It's that kind of heaviness where everything gets swelled up. It needs to be released and not held in the physical so much." She paused to take a long breath.

"And there's this frustration, the feeling symbolic, hitting your head on something. I can't get past this. Echoing. Pause and feel the actual pain of the experience, and that loss of her. Whoever you were before. She's you, but she's not. You're free to be whoever you are in this life. This will filter down. Stay warm in your blanket, in your cocoon," Kate sighed out. "I'm not going to open my eyes, or I'll lose my shit," she took another long breath.

"Your breath is on your side in this case. Shift some of it down through the roots. You're going to feel it in your solar plexus down to your sacral space. There's a lot of holding."

Kate continued to cry, and I did the same along with her. Bethan continued to hold space for the intimate healing experience.

"Ok. I should probably get a tissue or something. How are you doing? It's heavy. Not everyone has past life shit to deal with it," Kate said.

I nodded and wiped the tears from my eyes.

"I'm so interested in this past life thing," Bethan said. "I regressed someone recently and they went to a past life." Bethan was a hypnotherapist.

"Didn't I tell you that you and Bethan should connect more?" Kate asked.

"Yes," I agreed.

"I'm making a note to re-listen to my past life course and contact Aubree," Bethan announced.

"The past life things just come to me. I don't try to go there. Not everyone knows their past life experiences. Maybe if you need more detail than what I've given to you. It may help prove it to you. Seeing flashes of images may help you process it. You're going to feel this in your gut, in your sacral space. It's going to impact your heart. You're going to have to be powerful. You're going to have to be able to say that you're ready to let it go," Kate told me.

"It's a powerful day," I said. "Eclipse. Full moon. Letting go." They agreed.

"What are your plans are for the rest of the day?" Kate asked.

"Probably nothing now," I laughed.

"Do something grounding. Stimulate deep rest. Take a time out for quiet."

"Ok," I agreed.

"We did some major energy healing work on your head. It's like pieces of a puzzle coming back together. I keep seeing shards of light like glass coming back together. I tried to mend it together. I wish I could work on you in person."

"Me too," I said.

Kate reminded me that I was going to feel the impacts in my body, and to make rest a priority.

"Do you feel Ok? Do you feel safe?" she asked.

"Yes."

When I woke up the next day, I felt really fuzzy. I got up out of bed and lost my balance, falling right into the wall. I stumbled to the bathroom, then straight back to bed. I couldn't focus on anything. My brain felt scrambled.

What had happened? Powerful shifts in my head.

Both Kate and Bethan reached out to me to make sure I was okay. I told them both I was going back to bed. That's all I could do. I could barely sit up.

Bethan offered up a healing session to me. She was intrigued by the past life stuff, and wanted to work with me. I was feeling hopeful about this new avenue of exploration. After reading Dr. Weiss' book I felt inspired to have my own. Why not see what else was lurking in the shadows?

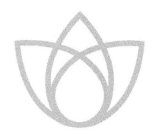

21. Letting Go

"We hang on to pain. It certainly satisfies our unconscious need
for the alleviation of guilt through punishment.
We get to feel miserable and rotten.
The question then arises, 'But for how long?'"

~ David R. Hawkins, Letting Go: The Pathway to Surrender

$\mathcal{A}$s part of Kate's mastermind group with me, Bethan had witnessed much of what Kate pulled from my energy field. As a hypnotherapist, she was curious to see if she could help with the endometriosis and infertility factors. I'd always wanted to do hypnosis, although I'd been a bit afraid about what would come up. What was hiding in my subconscious mind?

I was curious about the influence of past life memories and experiences, be that from my soul or ancestral imprints. After reading story after story of healing in *Miracles Happen*, I wondered if I could find success if I was witness to my own past memories. Up until that point it'd all be relayed to me through Kate's visions.

The emotions of it all, and connection to my chakra energy centers was profound. I couldn't deny everything that had come from these experiences.

On a Saturday morning chat with Bethan, she brought up her offer again, "We could do a session now if you're ready?"

Was I ready?

"Ok," I said, instinctively. I felt a turn in my solar plexus.

Bethan invited me to take a couple of long breaths with my eyes turned upwards towards my brain. This action was supposed to help bridge a physical connection to the subconscious.

She then guided me into a relaxed state, descending down, going deep into calm, deeper into myself, into old memories of the past. She asked me what I saw. What was the environment under my feet?

I was barefoot in the dirt. Overhead was a small shelter, like a hut.

"How do you feel?" she asked.

"Afraid," I answered.

I watched the images play out through my mind's eye, and the feelings of the encounter in my body. I felt anxious.

"Why are you afraid?" Bethan asked.

"I'm hiding," I paused. "I've been a bad girl." My words came out quiet. I was young, seven or eight years old. My heart raced as adrenaline pumped through me.

I was afraid of him.

The figure appeared at the entrance to the hut, towering above me. He pulled me by my long hair. I couldn't keep up with the momentum, and I fell to the ground, to my knees. I looked up at the night sky, and the trees of the forest. It was cold. I could see my breath. I felt a sharp pain on my right side as I was kicked there.

My vision was blurred when a rope slipped around my neck. I felt the pull — the drag of my body hitting the ground.

Bethan guided me to another memory. The scene was set at the opening of a cave on the edge of a mountainous ridge. I could hear the break of water below. I was dressed in a long dress that flowed behind me, as the wind whipped off the ocean.

"How do you feel?" she asked.

The same anxiety lived in my body, mixed with a deep sadness. I took a step to the edge of the cliff, then dove into the deep water below.

"What happened after you jumped into the water?"

"Nothing," I whispered. The life was gone. I jumped to my death, to the depths of the ocean, the element of the sacral space.

I killed myself. Death with impact of the water.

Bethan took me to one final memory. Fire burned around me, lighting the battle scene. I was a young boy running through the woods. I was afraid. Then, I was scooped up and thrown on the back of a horse by someone who brought me to a safe place where I got warm by the fire.

"That's the first time I've had a session where so many past life experiences came through," Bethan said after she pulled me back to the here and now.

Is that what they were? Did I actually experience those events? Where did those images come from? I couldn't deny the emotions from the experiences were strong.

A theme that showed in all these memories was a feeling of fear. I didn't feel safe. Bethan helped me define another soul lesson, and presence of a deeper fear, "I'm not safe." This subconscious belief vibrated under the surface.

When your body doesn't think it's safe, then subsequently it doesn't think it's safe to bring a baby into this world, and it naturally decreases progesterone levels. Cortisol, your stress hormone, competes with progesterone, which is necessary for pregnancy, and cortisol wins every time. That's because survival is your body's natural priority. When you're fearful and stressed, your body thinks you're in danger, releasing cortisol in response.

Another lesson that came through with Bethan was the purpose of pain as a reminder that I'm alive, that I'm really here in this body that my soul's been trying to escape from for much of my life. She explained how it was a common theme for those with chronic pain to have some sort of subconscious attachment to it.

Bethan gave me an audio to listen to everyday for the next 21 days where she guided me into a state of relaxation and presented positive truths. "Your voice matters. People listen to you. In the past, pain served as a way to remind you that you're alive, but it's no longer needed in this life..."

There were times when her words caused tears to flow out. On a deeper level, my soul self knew she spoke the truth.

I watched the music video for the Tori Amos song, *Horses*, as suggested by Kate to release "her", the past life energy who'd been strangled for expressing herself. I witnessed a similar experience in my session with Bethan. I could feel the burn around my neck. I was young, seven or eight. Was my soul re-living that trauma? I thought back to the night terrors that shook my world at that age.

I watched the first *Horses* music video to show up on YouTube which included images of connection between different women and horses. One was a woman laying on her back on the back of the horse, in surrender. Coupled with the music and Tori's beautiful voice, the tears came easily, along with a heavy ache in my heart and throat. It was time to let the pain from that experience go. It was time to forgive.

The issue of safety and security had shown up in exploration of my root chakra space, and it showed up again in past memories. With Bethan and Kate's help I'd uncovered underlying blocks and beliefs. Fear. I'm not safe. I needed pain to remind me that I'm alive.

A spiritual lesson presented itself. Could one be truly "safe" in this world? The vibration of fear's the backbone of American life. The media and corporations feed on it, especially the insurance companies. It was hard not to pick up on that. As an empath, honestly, I find the world to be overwhelming. It feels out of control, and really, it is.

The sacral chakra relates to the need to control the dynamics of your external life. According to Dr. Caroline Myss in the book *Anatomy of the Spirit*, illnesses that originate in the sacral chakra, like endometriosis, are activated by the fear of losing control.

Control. That was the fear I'd pinpointed when I first started digging into the influences of past energy. It came up as my greatest fear. *I'll lose control.*

The fear came from feeling a loss of power over my physical body. That was the feeling I knew far too well given the incredible amount of pain from endometriosis, a condition that felt out of control. I couldn't see it, I couldn't know what was going on inside.

When things started to feel out of control, when I felt anxious and unsafe, I made a shift and asked for help from greater spiritual entities that I trusted were there. I prayed to my angels and guides. This was greatly needed as the emotions poured out after my session with Bethan.

"I'm safe and protected." I found myself saying this aloud when fearful thoughts came up. I imagined a shield of light bubbling me, and an army of angels around me.

Releasing control to greater spiritual factors helped me calm down. My breath pulled me back into my body and settled my nervous system. Letting go of that which was out of my control released the tension in my body and mind.

As a result, I learned the biggest step towards *freedom*; it came with surrender. When negative emotions or stress rose up, I practiced feeling my way through them. I acknowledged how I was feeling. Rather than my typical running away mechanisms, I stayed present, without judgment.

When you simply live with the current sensation and acknowledge it, it loses its pull. You release suffering, which is resistance. Suffering is wanting things to be different from how they are now, but it can only be now, and there are painful moments when nothing works. All you can do is be with it.

Letting go is an act of acceptance of the situation as it is. It's not to surrender to your fears, but rather to see yourself as larger than the pain, larger than your body. This exercise of wholeness transcends your problems and starts to come naturally with regular practice. Nurture it as you breathe deep and release it. When you do this practice, resist judgment. Feel it as it is. Desires for things to be different from what they actually are is wishful thinking.

I connected with how I felt in my body and where certain emotions gathered. Sometimes I cried. Then I released it. There were times when I literally felt it go out of me. What a relief.

With this practice of surrender came another major shift. I opened up to receive. I stopped trying to control everything. I opened up for help and guidance, and when I verbally declared this, it came to me. This helped me to release old traumas that'd been stuck within my energy for nearly two decades, and further trauma that expanded beyond my physical existence in this body with endometriosis.

I believe there's a reason why the nervous system's so hyped up with endo. There's a reason why I've been so sensitive to everything. I've been forced to pay attention. It's time to receive. The message was presented to me many times along the way.

When I opened up to receive, the healing I needed came to me. When I opened up to receive, I created space for the pain to leave. When I opened up to receive, I connected with my intuition, and the messages and guidance from the divine.

My being open to receiving, helped return sex to an act of pleasure and greater soul connection with Ryan, my love and partner in this life, through endometriosis and whatever's next. Sex was happening much more often. How far we'd come in a year! I let go of the resistance in my sacral space that'd been held up by a thick wall of distrust. Sex with Ryan became amazing again. I felt love for my body that allowed me to experience the spiritual connection of orgasm and pure pleasure running through my physical existence. I deserved that, in this life, *now*.

It was as if I cracked wide open like the orange butterfly that continued to visit me under the sun. I'd finally broken *free*.

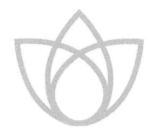

22. Mind/Body Connection

"I am willing to release the pattern within me that is creating this condition."

~ Louise Hay, You Can Heal Your Life

While I'd made huge strides on my healing journey with my periods and with sex, I still felt daily pain in my lower chakra areas. My lower back and hips ached most of the time. It was better when I stretched those areas out, or went for a massage, but that relief was short lived. I'd learned to cope with chronic pain in those areas, to a certain extent.

I wondered if there was more that I could do. On that excruciating day of pain a year before, when I finally reached out for help from Dr. Cook, and got the price of what surgery would cost, I learned that it was out of reach ... until it wasn't. My parents offered up the funds to pay for the surgery with a reminder that they wanted me to feel better and be able to have a family of our own. I no longer had anything holding me back.

Yet something did.

When I considered surgery, and the trauma that naturally came with that process, I felt a pull in my solar plexus. Cutting into my body didn't feel like the right thing to do. I thought back to the trauma the experience of surgery had on my body and how long it took to heal from that. Did I really want to go through that again?

I brought up the consideration of surgery in Kate's mastermind group. What should I do? My intuition said, "no", yet the external world continued to present excision surgery as *the* way of treating endometriosis. Was I crazy for not wanting to do that? Was this another test of me not trying hard enough?

The conversation in the mastermind group stemmed from discussion on the teachings of Louise Hay in her book, *Heal Your Body, Heal Your Life*. Louise taught on the connection between emotions, energy, and physical health. I'd seen that connection first hand, along with the powerful impacts of releasing old trauma and emotions. I'd personally experienced how energy work had helped release the pain from my periods, yet there was still pain that lingered. It was there physically, and I felt like that part still needed to be addressed.

"I need help," I said.

Those were words I didn't commonly share, but with my shifts in receiving, they fell in line.

Kate confirmed again that she would love to work on me in person. I could only imagine the magic that would bring. She lived on the other side of the country, however, so it wasn't going to happen right away.

In the meantime, my verbal declaration of receiving, "I need help", stimulated more synchronicity. I logged into Facebook and saw a post by a gal that I went to IIN with. She spoke of a new fascia release technique that had helped her finally release the chronic pain she'd struggled with for most of her life. I saw that while she was in Boulder recently, she had trained with her mentor, Elisha, who lived about an hour from me. I scoped out Elisha's web site and sent a message inquiring about the technique and endometriosis.

Elisha and I chatted a couple days after, and I was immediately drawn to her. I could tell that she was passionate about what she did. She'd found a way to help people with chronic pain find relief in a shorter period of time through her unique fascia release technique, which she'd coined as Kinetix.

Fascia is a band or sheet of connective tissue beneath your skin that's primarily made up of collagen. It's flexible and surrounds your muscles or other internal organs. Elisha described it as intelligent tissue that transmits communication to other nerves. It serves as a bridge between physical and emotional pain, a "wiring" of your nervous system response. Because of this connection, many people experienced emotional release with the treatment she did.

I told her about the pain I'd struggled with in the lower half of my body, my root. She said that the fascia in the lower back could impact pelvic alignment. Your abdomen and lower back are covered by a layer of fascia. It's right underneath your skin, and is the most pain-sensitive tissue in your body. It forms a body-wide network that communicates with itself like nerves do.

Elisha explained how stress and trauma to the gut cause adhesions to that area, resulting in a blockage of flow in your digestive tract. You also get adhesions from surgery. Every time you get cut open, your body's natural way to heal is with scar tissue, yet another reason why I wanted to avoid surgery. Scar tissue is primarily made up of collagen, just like the fascia that surrounds everything.

That scar tissue, combined with fascia, can envelope your insides like cobwebs, suffocating the normal blood flow and nutrition to the areas of your body. As a result, you feel stiffness, tightness, and pain. Chronic pain. Fascia needs space so that blood can flow.

Elisha felt confident that she could help me with the pain in my lower back and hips, so I scheduled an appointment. Her technique combined movement, and release of the fascia with her foot. The combined movement and pressure made me an active participant in the process.

Since the connection was between the physical and emotional link with the fascia, it was important to consciously have the mind/body link. This was different from other therapies like deep tissue massage, when the one receiving wasn't actively engaged in the release, nor had control over the movement.

Her office was about an hour away, located just outside my first college campus. The views on the drive up reminded me why I went to school there. I felt a tug at my heart space as I pulled into the old familiar territory, and the feelings of fear the memories held.

On my first day in the dorm room I remembered being greeted with a welcome letter, a map of campus, and a silver whistle attached to a red cord. I picked it up for closer review. There was a police symbol etched into the side. My eyes moved to the slip of paper under the shiny object. The whistle was to be used in an emergency. There'd been attacks on campus, more so than most college campuses in the country.

It was a rape whistle.

As an incoming freshman, I had a last pick of classes. I was also near last on the list when it came to parking. I had to park my car in a lot that was miles away, and take a bus back to my building. The bus dropped off in designated locations, and mine was quite a bit away from my dorm room. I didn't feel safe walking late nights on the path lined with emergency call stations. I held my rape whistle tight in hand, worried that I would be attacked and violated.

One night while my roommate and I slept, the door to our dorm room opened. I woke up from the bright light in the hallway, and in a half-dream state, watched a large man walk in. He reeked of alcohol. His body wavered in the area between our beds. We both sat up. I held the blankets tight, my knees bent up in defense, as fear coursed through my body. Where was my whistle?

We watched in shock as he gave a goofy grin, with unrecognizable words that ended with his body folding to the floor. My roommate looked at me with wide eyes.

I still had the blankets close to my chest. There was no getting out of the bed without having to step over him. That felt vulnerable, given my bare legs and tiny bedtime shorts. My imagination was fueled with years of horror film scenes. He'd grab my ankle. He'd pull me down. He was a big dude with thick muscles and he was clearly heavily intoxicated, which made him unpredictable.

We didn't know what to do, so we sat and waited. My eyes scanned the room. My bed was pushed up against the wall and I was blocked in at the end by a desk. There was no other way out. The room felt like a trap.

I watched his body and waited for signs of movement. Then he started to snore. My roommate called for help and campus security carried the drunken man out of our room, though he forgot to take my fear with him. The incident stimulated a triple check every time I shut the door, to ensure that it was locked. I no longer felt the sense of freedom from being away at college. I felt unsafe. The following semester I decided to move back home.

The memories filled my consciousness as I drove onwards to Elisha's office, where I was to make another step to release those old emotions from the physical part of my body. Those emotions vibrated with a consistency of fear and an old belief that, *"I'm not safe"*.

"Your fascia holds an imprint of your whole life," Elisha explained.

She focused treatment primarily on the lower part of my body. She was able to pick up on the memories that still lived in my fascia. She could even tell that I played soccer as a kid.

I smiled at the memory, "I liked to kick the ball hard," I told her. I enjoyed playing in the front-line positions where I had a chance to score. Even back then I was competitive.

"Everyone's different when it comes to your stress response,"

Elisha explained. She picked up on patterns as she worked with people and how they responded to the treatment.

"Some people are wired for more intensity, which means that you can handle a lot more pain."

Having lived through the hell of endometriosis, I knew all about pain. The pain that she brought during the fascia release exercises was nothing in comparison. Yes, the release hurt at times, but I didn't show it.

"I have a high pain tolerance," I said.

"Me too. I'm wired for intensity, which means that I stay around too long in situations that don't serve me because I think that I can handle it," Elisha said.

I understood and could relate. There was a difference between her and me though. She saw it in the way I responded. After each position and release she asked me how I felt. Did I feel any different?

"I don't know," I said.

"How do you feel now?" Elisha asked again.

"Better, I guess," I said. The sensation in my legs was strange, but I couldn't tell if it was better.

"How do you feel now?" she asked again.

I found myself getting frustrated when she asked the question.

"You're detached," she observed.

She wasn't the first to point that out. My soul has been trying to escape for a long time. That was understandable given the amount of pain my body brought.

"It's a defense mechanism," I admitted.

"Absolutely."

Her words stuck with me because they were a reminder of what I'd learned, and what still needed to expand — my roots. I needed to make an effort to come back into my body and experience the sensations of life. Movement helped with that. Getting outside with earthly connection, getting creative, having sex. I needed to do more of these things and enjoy my existence in this body I lived in. Yes, it brought pain, but it was also capable of experiencing joy.

Elisha granted me with further belief that it's possible to live in a body without pain. She'd seen it again and again from people who'd pretty much given up on the idea. I walked away with a spark of hope.

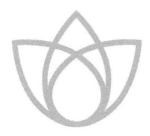

23. The Fire Burns

"I am that I am."

Exodus 3:14

*A*t this point I was fully aware of how powerful energy work was. I could feel physical shifts in my body, as the horrible pain with my periods stayed away.

My curiosity and positive experience with Audra and Reiki intrigued me enough to study that, too. I soon saw that what I learned in the Reiki course was only a fraction of what I'd learned from Kate, but I did take away some tidbits to expand what I'd been doing. Reiki helped me become more hands on as I tuned into my different chakra areas.

My Reiki attunement was scheduled at 2:20 on August 22nd. The twos. Ever since I connected with the Goddess Hathor in *The Sophia Code*, the twos showed up all the time, at the perfect time. Hathor's message is all about receiving and expression. She relates to the throat space. Her Sophia code of "two" continued to show up in my life, so it seemed the perfect time to receive my attunement.

A Reiki attunement is a powerful spiritual experience where energies are channeled into the student through the Reiki master. The attunement I received was done at a distance. I'd learned from working with Kate that you don't have to be in the same room with someone to connect with them energetically. You pick up vibes. Everything is energy and it interacts, regardless of space.

When the time arrived, I popped on my headphones, sat back in my black papasan chair, and pulled in the meditative music. The experience was powerful. I felt a strong pressure at my third eye, and the transfer of energy down my entire chakra system. I had a strong visualization of an elephant being bitten by a bunch of mosquitoes. I felt almost paralyzed, as I did during a normal Reiki session.

It's said that attunement can increase psychic sensitivity. It can also cause a detox reaction, as the energy moves up old stuff. I felt that for sure. I was tired, grumpy, and super out of it for the next few days.

Following my attunement, I had a dream that I was in my parent's room in the house I grew up in, and the phone started to ring. It was one of the old school corded versions with the heavy receiver and big buttons. My grandmother's voice sounded on the other end, clear as day, just as I remembered it. It startled me enough to wake me up.

It was suggested that after receiving Reiki energy, you practice on yourself every day for at least three weeks. So, the next day I settled on my back on the couch with a blanket over me to do just that. As usual, I put on my headphones and closed my eyes, falling into the rhythm of the meditative music, and placing my hands in position as I'd learned through the Reiki training.

I was called to my sacral space. I placed my hands right below my belly button and continued to take long and deep breaths, bringing attention to this part of my body, falling into a deeply relaxed state. I did a scan of my body and felt the familiar pain on my right side. It was throbbing. I moved my palm over the pain at the curve of the back of my pelvic bone and asked a silent question; *why is this pain here?*

In my mind's eye, I saw an image of a snake, uncoiling. As my body sunk into even deeper relaxation, I saw a clear visual of a baby, sitting in a carrier on the ground by itself. Then, a big black sword sliced across my vision, cutting in front of my view of the small child. I felt a strong pulsing in my sacral space. I moved my hands to my belly as I felt the movement of energy rise up, as if I was pulling out a ball of energy. I lifted it from my sacral space and a flood of emotions poured out of my closed eyes until I was sobbing.

Something big released — I felt it.

I looked up the meaning of the snake in my *Pocket Guide to Spirit Animals*, and my mouth dropped open when I read the meaning. *"You're about to go through some significant personal changes, so intense and dramatic that an old self will metaphorically die as a new self emerges... you're about to resolve a long-standing issue, one that has required a great deal of your attention, by seeing things in a new light... you'll experience a dramatic and unexpected physical or emotional healing very soon, coming from an unexpected source."*

I mentioned the experience to Kate and the other ladies in the mastermind call. What was that all about?

"You took care of whatever needed to go there," Kate said.

I think she was right. Perhaps the vision was a way for my subconscious to cut that cord and allow true healing to occur. I was taken aback, yet again, by the power within me. It'd been recognized and put to use in a big way. I'd made a difference on myself. I think the unexpected source was *me*. I took a moment to soak that in.

I practiced doing energy readings on myself, and on the other ladies in the group, and found myself getting better at picking up on images and messages in the energy field. It was helpful to work with Kate and the others to confirm that they received similar messages. That helped to grow my confidences in what I felt and intuitively knew.

I was ready to step out of the safety of the small mastermind group and practice on other women in the Peace with Endo community. I reached out to see if there were any ladies that would be willing to let me practice doing energy readings and chakra balancing, and I got a few volunteers.

I was nervous to do my first reading on my own, but I swallowed the fear and moved forward. The main concern of the first woman I worked on was a lack of sex drive. The issue made me immediately think of the sacral space, and the imbalance of giving and receiving. My intuition told me that she was likely giving more than receiving, and the energy was showing up in her pelvic area.

My instinct was spot on. She hadn't been making time for herself or space for self-care. As an entrepreneur, she put a lot of pressure on herself, and as a result, she worked long hours.

As soon as I tuned into her energy, I felt a throbbing at my throat.

"I'm feeling some tension in the throat area," I said, as I cleared mine.

"You can? Wow. I've been having issues with my throat for the past few months."

She'd had a viral infection, and was recently diagnosed with an underactive thyroid. She was amazed that I could pick up on that. I walked her through some breathing exercises to help clear the throat area, as I'd seen Kate do to me before.

"I feel better," she said.

I felt a stirring in her sacral space, so we did some breath work there, too.

"Make sure you're making space to receive," I said. "Schedule yourself in. It's necessary that you take care of you."

She agreed that she needed to make that shift.

"Express yourself," I said, as I cleared my throat again. "I'm still feeling tension there."

I walked her through another set of breathing exercises with verbal release out of the mouth.

"How do you express yourself creatively?" I asked.

"I like to sing," she said.

"Perfect," I smiled. "Do that tonight and as much as you can in the days to come."

After the call with her, my throat continued to throb, and I started to freak out a bit. I'd picked up on her energy in a big way, so I reached out to Kate, who reminded me to be sure I grounded and protected myself before my calls. I hadn't taken enough time to do that.

I laughed out loud later that night when realization hit. The answers I needed to heal my own throat came in mirroring effect, yet again; the advice I gave to my client was what I needed to heed for myself. I needed to create space for rest, fun, and creative expression. It was necessary. I sang the song Kate sent me before, "See the sun..."

I took a break in the mid-afternoon sun. It was hot. I sat on my reclining chair with a book I'd been loving on called *White Hot Truth*, by Danielle LaPorte. I could relate to her words and appreciated her underlying message that you have to find your own truth. It's not up to some guru — it's up to you.

I couldn't stay outside for long. The air filled up with smoke. Fire, something was burning. It made me rise up from my lounge chair to make sure the yard next to ours wasn't on fire. I could see a pour of smoke through the crack in the fence from the makeshift fire pit next door. I looked around but didn't see anyone.

I went back inside, but the fear of the smoke didn't leave me. It was dry out, and fires had been burning up the state. There was a fire ban in effect, and for good reason. One little ember and it could all go up in flames. Both of our yards were dry from lack of water. What if it all burned down?

Worry took over me. I expressed my concern to Ryan, whose

unease only added to my own. I checked back on the flames every ten minutes or so to make sure they hadn't caught on anything.

My fear drove me to call the police. I was afraid. As soon as I did this, the fire went out on its own, and I felt a little silly.

The fire and smoke in the summer sky reminded me of the story of Moses in the book of Exodus. Deeper meaning in this story was relayed within the book *The Moses Code*, by James F Twyman.

Moses was an Israelite slave. According to the law set forth by the Egyptian Pharaoh, every male child born to Israelite slaves was to be drowned in the Nile. In fear of the repercussions that would come from Moses' birth, his mother set her infant son adrift on the Nile in a small craft. A short distance down the river, the Pharaoh's daughter found the baby and adopted him as her son. She named him Moses, meaning "to draw out". Due to divine intervention he was raised a prince.

The story continues when Moses is a man and brave leader of the Egyptian empire. One day as he as leading his flock up Mount Horeb, he saw a bush that burned with bright fire, yet the fire didn't consume it. It's here that Moses meets God in physical form for the first time, in symbolism of fire.

God called to him from the bush and said, "Moses, Moses."

And Moses said, "Here I Am." (Ex 3:4). He didn't run away with fear.

Hearing this response, it's as if God is pleased.

"Do not draw away. Take your shoes from your feet, for the place where you stand is holy ground." (Ex 3:5)

The place was holy because it was the spot where God manifested into this world.

The Moses Code theorized that the ground was holy because it was the spot where Moses came in touch with his true Self. God was pleased because Moses seemed to recognize himself as one with his Creator.

God told Moses that he was to lead the Israelites out of Egypt. When Moses asked who he should say sent him with this message, God spoke a powerful set of words, *"I am that I am."*

According to *The Moses Code*, these words were the greatest gifts God has ever given to humanity, for the secret to creating miracles was revealed. These words indicate the truth that God is within you. You are a divine creation, and because of that, you have the ability to heal.

The fire had been a recurring theme in my life, and within my explorations towards *freedom*. Once I began learning about the chakras, I saw this symbol connecting back to personal power, and how this related to every energetic disturbance that had happened since.

I'd lost my power along the way, lifetimes ago, but I was ready to step into it. My soul had opened up and truth was revealed. I was powerful beyond measure. I had the ability to implement change and take action. I was finally aware of my personal power.

Following my fear of the smoke and fire next door, I sat outside under the glow of the summer evening dusk with my dogs, Alice and Einstein. Einstein was next to me. His butt wiggled, the epitome of joy. He loved the sound of my laughter. It made his butt wiggle even more, which made me giggle even more. Before I knew it, I was cracking up, in a good way.

This came in line with my own awareness cracking open. I saw that moment of pure bliss that the true me was in the presence of joy.

That didn't mean that life wasn't a struggle sometimes, but those were passing emotions. They weren't the real me they were like the storm clouds passing through.

In that moment, under the night sky that glowed with a reflection of the sun, I laughed. Einstein wiggled and let out his boxer voice, his song. Together we danced under the moonlight in pure presence of joy.

When we build walls and protection, that energy isn't able to flow freely. I'd broken down many of them. Once I got through the grief, I felt more expansive, and in alignment with my soul. The wall that released in my pelvic space brought down the walls during sex, which was happening with Ryan more frequently.

I found myself fully present in the act, and when I tuned into the merge of energy in a beautiful dance of soul connection, I released the struggle, trusted and connected to the shared spiritual energy that came from an intimate act. It served as a way to ground my body and stimulate that sacral energy, and it sure relieved a lot of tension in our household.

I felt a vibration at my heart. I literally opened up to receive. The energy in my sacral space was flowing again, along with its earthly connection to water. The natural lubrication helped a lot with sex. I felt the waves of pleasure.

The Wild Woman was rising. She was finally free. I was a goddess.

Ryan repeated my thought aloud as our sexual energy intertwined, "You're a goddess."

I smiled in silent knowing of our intuitive connection in an act that was full of pleasure and love. I was worth it, and finally receiving it.

I closed my eyes, and a dragon appeared in my mind's eye. I smiled wider. I was powerful beyond measure. I finally realized it. My sacral energy flowed again.

There's no more fear of the fire, I know now that it is part of me, burning powerful inside.

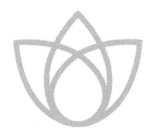

24. Expect Miracles

"There are only two ways to live your life.
One is as though nothing is a miracle.
The other is as though everything is a miracle."

~ Albert Einstein

Ryan and I returned from a short trip out of town. A wave of disquiet washed over me. I felt lost, overwhelmed, and anxious. The plane trip home was long and especially uncomfortable for Ryan, whose tall frame didn't fit well into the compacted space of an airplane. A couple with two young children sat behind us. The baby was very vocal. He sat on the lap of his father right behind Ryan's seat. Every so often Ryan felt the rattling kick of the baby's foot into his spine.

After the fifth kick or so Ryan turned around and asked the parents if they could help settle the young boy's flailing legs. The interaction seemed to trigger something deeper, a kick from the universe of what was missing from our lives.

By the time we hit the ground we were both exhausted. I'd picked up on the energy from the experience in a big way, feeling the anxiety course through me mixed with sadness. I needed to come back to my own energy. Since being away, I hadn't taken the time to meditate, and I had little to no alone time.

I was happy to be home. I settled into my regular routine; earphones, papasan chair, eyes closed. I grounded and protected myself, and recited my openness to receive.

"Please give me a sign. I need guidance. Angels. Please," I whispered.

During the meditation, I saw a clear face of a hawk in my third eye. Then I saw a buffalo.

When I opened my eyes, Ryan appeared in the front room. The dogs were there too, their stance alert, as they stood looking out the front window. They were interested in something in the yard.

"What is it?" Ryan asked, as he looked out the front window with them. "Whoa!"

"What is it?" I repeated.

"There's a big 'ol hawk on the fence!"

I got up to see, to confirm what I'd just seen in my mind, a clear vision of a hawk. I'd never seen one that close before. I marveled at the large wings on the bird as he fluffed them up. I watched as it lifted off from the fence, soaring up into the air. There was magic alive in that moment. I could feel it.

I asked for a sign, saw a hawk in my meditation, and one appeared outside at the same time. I took it as a message from spirit, and reminder of the power of my intuition and innate energetic field.

I went down to pick up my Spirit Animal guide book and turned to the "H's" for Hawk. The following passage send a wave of goose bumps through me, *"Pay close attention to your surroundings, as you're about to receive an important message."*

I flipped back to the "B's" to look up the image of the buffalo I'd received. The passage I found there summed up an important message. I share it with you now, because it sums up this story, and my perspective on living a life with endometriosis and related infertility. It relates to an unknown future of what may or may not happen, and to those days that you feel down and out, lost, overwhelmed, sad. It's also pretty straight up advice that I needed at the time.

*"Focus on being appreciative and grateful for all that you have.
Have faith in the natural abundance of life.
Stop feeling sorry for yourself and instead be aware of the extraordinary
number of resources you have available....
Expect a miracle and keep the faith."*

~ Dr. Steven Farmer, Pocket Guide to Spirit Animals

Ryan and I settled into a corner booth in the restaurant. It was a Saturday night that I'd spent putting finishing touches on this story.

The restaurant wasn't one that we frequented often since its menu was pricey. We'd been there a couple of times on celebratory occasions like my birthday. We were there that day because we'd received a complementary meal in the mail, and because we were both starving. Big surprise.

We were placed next to a family who had a small child. Every so often the little girl would let out a shriek that made my entire nervous system stand on edge. I could tell from Ryan's flinches that it did the same to him.

I took a look at the mother, and saw the exhaustion lined on her face. I felt a tug of compassion at my heart space. I bet it was hard to be a mother of a young child. I wondered when was the last time she had a full night sleep, or an hour to herself to do what she wanted?

Like I could. I had the freedom to do what I wanted with my time. *Freedom*. I took a moment to be grateful for that, and more so when the family left the restaurant along with the horrible shrieks of that little girl. I took a moment of gratitude for the return of peace and connection with Ryan's baby blue eyes.

There are ups and downs in the journey of grieving from infertility, but there is truth to the statement that it gets easier with time. I accept the fact that there will always be an ache in my heart, of a loss in the past, and one of an idea of what could have been. When those feelings of sadness rose up, I allowed them to flow through, so that they can pass through, and I could return to the higher vibrations in the present moment of love and joy.

I see now that while I haven't been able to create new life, I can still create in other ways. I can still stimulate my natural motherly instinct. Even without the fruit of new life, I embrace the power of creation that's within me, and with that I birth love into this world through my words, through my music, and by sharing my voice.

Creativity is healing. It's in direct energetic alignment with the power of creation within you, the power of creation that *is* you. Acts of creation grant a direct pathway to your higher Self. Through these acts, I was helping the world. I helped women who were in pain. Since I didn't have a child, I had more time for that.

A bigger vision started to form in my mind, stimulated by a growing force from the divine feminine energy that'd been rising within me for months. If I could help heal women in the world, what an impact I could have!

"I do have something to celebrate today," I said.

"What's that?" Ryan asked.

"Five years ago today, I published my first post on my blog at peacewithendo.com." I smiled remembering how scared I was to share my voice with the Internet. It started out anonymous as simply "Peace with Endo". Then I added my first name, and finally my last name. There was no more hiding the fact that I had endometriosis. As a result of putting my voice out there, I'd connected with amazing women from around the world. Peace with Endo had gone from my weekly blog project to a full out worldwide movement. It was something to celebrate.

"Is something burning out there?" I asked.

My side of the booth faced a wall of windows. I noticed a band of smoke constantly floating up into the late summer sky.

Ryan turned around and stood up to see if he could see the source of the smoke.

"I don't know where that's coming from," he said.

As the meal progressed my eyes kept catching on the consistent billow of smoke. My curiosity made me stand up and take a closer look out the window. I couldn't see the source either. Maybe someone was smoking? It didn't make sense.

When we finished up and went to leave the restaurant, Ryan paused before pulling the car all the way out.

"Something is burning over there," he said. He paused in front of the source of the smoke; a bush that lined the parking lot.

Ryan reversed the car and I jumped out to take a look. I couldn't see where the source of the smoke came from, but something was on fire. I could smell the burning embers. I tried to stomp it out with my sneaker, but it didn't help.

Ryan went inside to let the staff in the restaurant know about the burning bush. I sat and contemplated the signal.

"God? Is that you?" I joked with Ryan on our drive home.

Isn't it ironic? Maybe. Synchronicity. There are no accidents. The burning bush was a reminder of that message, "I *am* that I *am*."

There is a fire inside and it burns bright. The light is your central fire that houses your personal power. Take a hold of it, love. What are you waiting for?

I believe that women with endometriosis are powerful. Your body is sensitive and receptive. The lesson is one on receiving. Your body is ready for it, all you have to do is open up and allow it to flow to you. Pay attention. You're being guided all the time. Once I opened up and allowed help and spiritual guidance to come in, I was directed to a grand path of healing and understanding. No matter how hard things get, no matter how hopeless it seems, you're never alone. There's greater guidance out there, and it's working in your favor. There are miracles happening every day.

You in yourself are a miracle, simply because of your existence.

You are made of love and light. I know it can be hard to see that sometimes. It took me a long time to understand that, living in a body that felt broken, that wasn't well enough to bring a new life into this world.

Once you truly see this, when you connect with it and realize the true beauty of your being, you too will find your way to *freedom*.

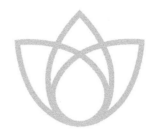

25. Energetics of Endo

*"If we stay aware and acknowledge the great mystery that is life,
we will see that we have been perfectly placed, in exactly the
right position... to make all the difference the world."*

~ James Redfield, The Tenth Insight: Holding the Vision

I remember that woman from the beginning of this story, the one with a deep ache in her heart space from what felt like a missing piece of the puzzle ... and I barely recognize her. She has transformed. I'm not the same woman I was.

Things shifted for me when I set an intention based on how I wanted to feel: *freedom*. Declaring my desire to feel *free* lead me down a path of greater spiritual growth, one I was not expecting, that evolved with freedom on a grander scale. It developed within, and expanded the more I let go.

I always felt like there was more to the story. Why did I suffer each menstrual cycle with horrible pain and contractions that I imagined were like labor pains, only to come away with a deep feeling of grief and emptiness? The experiences were traumatic, and caused constant anxiety and stress about the arrival of my period. It was a serious disruption in my life, but it also served as a forced awakening. The amount of pain left little other choice than to surrender, which turned out to be the best thing I could do on my path to *freedom*.

I couldn't deny the impacts the energy work had on my body and mind. As a result of the great amount of healing I'd received, the physical pain with my periods dropped away. They became mild, as I imagined a "normal" period is for most women. While there was still discomfort, it wasn't traumatic like it used to be.

Life with endometriosis felt more manageable. I waited for the pain with my periods to return, but it didn't. As the months of mild periods added up to a full year, I started to relax a little. I could tell that the trauma from the experience was gone. When pain did rear its head, I had the tools to manage it, and the power within to influence how I felt physically and emotionally. I took flare ups as a sign that I needed to slow down and rest.

I became aware of the workings of my mind space. I'm no longer a prisoner to my own thoughts or negative beliefs. I recognized that I had a choice in how I responded, and that response is my greatest power. When I lingered on certain negative thoughts or beliefs, I was only feeding my own suffering. As the saying goes, "Pain is inevitable. Suffering is optional."

I practiced pulling myself away from the thoughts that ruled my mind and back to the present moment. I started being more mindful, living life within sensations that are electrified outside of this realm of thought: the warmth of the sun on my skin, the feel of my feet on the ground, the tickle of the wind across my face, the joy from a good round of laughter, the ache from a good cry. I felt through the seasons, soaking it all in, learning to love the experiences in my body.

I understood the influence of my energy system and how the messages I've been relayed all contributed to the experience of my soul in a physical existence, in a body with endometriosis. Through the chakra system, I've learned so much about my Self, my body, and the part energy plays in physical and mental health. Because all of this information can be a little overwhelming, I've summarized the knowledge I've come to understand about the body's energy centers. I'm starting from the top down, since, unknowingly, that's how my journey evolved.

CROWN CHAKRA

The crown chakra, which sits right above the top of your head, is there to receive messages from source, angels, and guides. It's the space where spiritual awareness and intuitive guidance come through.

As I traveled down this energetic journey, I was told over and over again that my crown chakra was wide open. I think that was because I set a daily intention, verbally declaring that I was open to receiving, and taking at least ten minutes after to meditate. Meditation is the best way to receive these messages. Get quiet.

Once I made this intention of receiving part of my daily practice, things started to happen in synchronicity. I connected with the right people who helped me find healing on a deeper level. Information and opportunities came into my life in perfect timing.

Opening up to receive expanded my awareness of the presence of angels and guides. I found great comfort in knowing that I was always safe and protected.

THIRD EYE CHAKRA

The third eye chakra's located between your eyes at the pituitary gland, and is all about listening to and trusting your intuition. This is so important when it comes to healing. Trust that small voice inside. It always knows what's best for you.

With endometriosis we are offered different hormonal treatment options. Many times, these are presented as the only option. Please know that's not true! It's important to understand that all of these hormonal treatments manipulate your brain, primarily your pituitary gland, which is the conductor of your endocrine system, and the center of your third eye chakra. Once I released myself from the hormonal manipulation of birth control pills, I started to think more clearly. I felt more like myself. My intuition woke up.

The third eye relates to the power of your thoughts. A big shift happened when I had a conscious understanding that there was a distinct separation between the thoughts in my head, and the "witness" to these thoughts. That witness equates to my higher Self, my true Self, my soul. This true Self is divine and part of something greater, encompassing true love and a connection to creation.

I think that as humans our natural underlying desires are to be seen, loved, acknowledged, and understood. That can be hard when you have a chronic illness, or when you develop in an environment when these attributes may be missing. What I've learned from my higher Self is that I'm already loved, acknowledged, and understood simply because of my being. Your being is naturally connected to love and light. You are not alone. You are seen. You are loved. You are whole. You don't need to look outward for confirmation of this. The truth is within. I promise you, it's all inside. With inner freedom comes greater outward experience.

One way to connect to your higher Self is through creative acts. When you create, you go to a different subconscious level. Do it every day you can. Connect with your higher Self and see what it has to say. You will find your way.

If you need more help finding your way, look to the mirroring effect that happens in your life, especially within your relationships. What lessons are being presented to you? Are you listening? Are you paying attention?

THROAT CHAKRA

The throat chakra is all about speaking your truth, sharing, and letting go. I've come away with awareness that my throat space is the primary area that needs attention. It's the area that's thrown the rest of my energy system out of whack.

It's time to find my voice. I've been the quiet girl, silenced early on by the bullies, violated and disregarded when I spoke up about the pain I experienced in my sacral space. My throat space held past woundings from speaking up and having others not like what I had to say. I see this fear pop up often in my life.

As a natural people pleaser, it's easier to stay quiet. I don't like to rock the boat. I've never liked standing out. Yet the lesson on speaking up forced its way into my existence. The horrible pain that came along with endometriosis shook me up. It made me want to scream.

I feel on purpose within the endo community of women that have also felt unheard. In sharing my story, I give rise to the energy of a cause that needs a voice, a positive voice. I've been drawn to this and I'm stepping into it. I do believe it's what I'm here to do. Use my voice.

I encourage you to do the same. Express yourself. You have the power to make change. Speak up. Share your story. Create art. Let's raise the vibe.

Heart Chakra

Your heart space is all about unconditional love. This starts with yourself. Self-love is what makes changes stick, and pulls you through when you want to quit. It's the whispered reminder in your ear that you deserve to feel better. Unconditional love has the greatest power of all. It's the instinct within you, the very nature of the life energy that flows through you. We all have that same vibrational energy of love inside.

It takes inner self-courage and acceptance to face the fear, but when you overcome it you become more capable and free. The way to overcome the fear is to surrender to it. Only then can you let it go, and experience your true nature. Rather than be governed by fear, you can instead choose love. Love vibrates at a higher energy than fear, overcoming it. Love is capable of healing, transforming, and enlightening.

When you let go of fear and replace it with love, you elevate your own consciousness. Could you not instill the same motivation or behavior out of love, rather than out of fear or guilt? Care, appreciate, and value your body with love, not out of fear of disease. Your body wants to find balance, but it needs your love and nurturing care.

When you become aware of the love inside of you, it grows stronger and you'll feel lighter. Finding the truth of who you really are will set you free. Being free from guilt creates space for renewed life energy. Your heart space is connected physically and energetically to your sacral space, which is all about creativity.

Look inside and find that innate innocence, the little girl who was the light, before the shadows crept in. Connect with her and you'll stop fighting with yourself, bullying yourself, or invalidating your worth. Be the love you wish you'd received during those dark times.

Offer up forgiveness. This is an offering of love to yourself. Let it go.

The heart space is also where your purpose lies. Are you on point with what stimulates excitement? What does your heart have to say? Create space to listen and take action.

Solar Plexus

The solar plexus, located at your navel, is your power center. You've been exploring this relationship to power ever since you were young, learning who had the power, how to attract it, and how to use it. The people in your life, and the choices you make each moment, are expressions and symbols of your personal power. If you learned along the way that you were only going to survive through the energies of other people, instead of using your own power, you may have an unbalanced view.

That imbalance can turn into a desire for power which can show up as addictions and cravings. For me, it led to an overachieving drive that burnt me out, literally. I thought I earned power by achieving external validation. Without an internal sense of power, external demands of material items become more appealing, or you become more prone to listening to outside authorities instead of the messages of your internal guidance.

You may hesitate to challenge someone who you believe holds more power than you, or may agree to do things because you don't believe you have the power to refuse. What gives you power or makes you feel powerless? Are you being controlled by an external power? Your solar plexus is where the establishment of healthy boundaries reigns. This is a big deal for my fellow empaths out there.

Your solar plexus is physically connected with your third eye via the vagus nerve. They work in tandem. If you're to follow your intuitive guidance, you must have the courage and personal power to follow through.

The concept of personal power in the solar plexus region shows up symbolically as fire, an inner flame that will not be extinguished by outer forces. The fire burns in reminder of what's possible. If you're going to get better, you must believe it's possible. You must believe in yourself. Low self-esteem reflects a lack of faith in yourself as one of the most powerful beings in the unseen world.

Sacral Chakra

Your sacral chakra is the one most influenced by endometriosis, and one that's governed by a fear of losing control. That comes with feelings of loss of power over your physical body. Both are feelings I understood with endometriosis and infertility. The lesson in the sacral space is that you can't always control the outside environment, but you do have a say in how you respond internally with your thoughts and emotions. The challenge of the sacral chakra is to learn what motivates you to make the choices that you make. Are you filled with fear, or with faith?

This becomes clear through the relationships in your life. They can bring revelation to your strengths and weaknesses. The patterns of energy generated in this space attract people who are opposite of you in some way, who have something to teach you, or help you come to know yourself. Relationships are the best way to see the mirroring effect in action. This showed up in my relationship with Ryan. We had plenty to teach each other. We were opposites in many ways, but these opposing forces balanced each other out.

There's a dual nature that's active in the sacral chakra. This division of forces shares different names: yin/yang, masculine/feminine, shadow/light, sun/moon. It encompasses the balance of giving and receiving. This dual nature challenges you to make choices in a world of opposing sides, of positive and negative energy patterns. It's all about balance.

The shadow side of the sacral chakra holds some of the strongest fears of rape, betrayal, abandonment, isolation, and the inability to care for your Self. Sexual violations in the form of rape, incest, and child molestation, are physical and energy violations motivated by another's desire to place control over you. These actions can leave behind heavy energetic scars that can also impact the physical organs in this space.

Violations in your sacral space aren't always physical. They can show up anytime another desires to cripple your ability to be independent and thrive outside the control of another person. Consistent criticism about your professional skills, ambitions, accomplishments, or your physical appearance, energetically violates your sense of personal power. Your sexual organs house these negative beliefs and emotions.

Your sacral charka is connected physically and energetically to your throat chakra and modes of expression. Within that throat and sacral connection, you learn to communicate in relationships and to express what you do or don't desire. We don't always learn how to express what we need sexually, which can lead to dissatisfaction from both parties, and can threaten the nature of your relationships. Worry about betrayal rises up, bringing more stress to this space.

The sacral space contains the desire and ability to birth new life. This happens through the spiritual act of sex, which serves as an avenue of self-expression in which you drop your physical boundaries in order to enjoy true pleasure. I know for many of us with endometriosis, this act can bring pain, but it doesn't have to be that way. When you release the tension in this area physically and emotionally, then pleasure wins. (There are hands-on therapies that can help release the tension including pelvic floor therapy and Maya massage.)

The sacral space is all about creativity, or the physical sensation of being alive. Creativity is a spiritual act in and of itself. The act of creation is one of the divine. With this creative energy comes a pull to release the past and find a new reason to move forward, even when challenges seem overwhelming. The energies of your sacral chakra bring up memories that need to be released. When you do, you pave the way to become more whole in body, mind, and spirit.

The sacral space is the energy center for the divine feminine, the Wild Woman, Sophia. If you feel lost, get back in the flow, connect to Mother Nature. Connecting back to nature's flow helps to re-align. Get outside. Go hang out by the trees, a river, lake, or ocean. Get out under the stars. Breathe in the outside air. Allow the divine feminine energy to illuminate your being. Put your feet flat on the ground, walk in the sand, the water, the grass.

Your body is restrictive. It comes with aches and pains, stabbings and sludge, but outside the weight of your skin, on a deeper spiritual level, you are unbounded and connected to everything. I didn't truly recognize this until I made it through the mud. I've always loved the connection with the lotus flower - no mud, no lotus. The lotus must pull through the mud and sludge to see the light. It's easier to find the light when you get in the sacral energy of creation. Connect with your soul power.

Root Chakra

The root chakra located at the base of your spine is the support for your entire energy system. If this space is off, it impacts all the others. The root space is complex and deep, as the root of the earth is. It enfolds deeper ancestral energy, fear, and feelings of alienation. After exploring the issues in my own root, it was clear to me I needed more support and understanding, as I'm sure most of my endo sisters do. Living with a chronic illness and/ or infertility can be isolating. It's important to cultivate positive support around you.

Connecting to the earth supports your root chakra space. It's a reminder of the support that's all around you, all the time. Love and honor this connection with gratitude and respect for the connection between your body, soul, and all things. Respect your body and the earth. Avoid the chemical disrupters that only encourage stagnation. Eat foods that come from the earth.

The roots and sacral space are connected by water. Water is the element of this space, so being around it, or in it, helps. This boundless connection with the entire earth and beyond is a collective creation that's happening in magical symphony all around you.

In order for me to truly find peace with endo, a spiritual shift was needed. With this came a strong knowing that no matter what happened, no matter how bad things got, I always made it through. Things always had a way of working themselves out.

While I'd love to leave this story with the perfect ending, of a child in my arms, the truth is it hasn't happened, and I'm not sure that it's going to. What I do know is that it's out of my hands. I surrender to what is. If this is indeed the end of the line, if no child is to be born of my womb, I'm grateful that I still get to spend this life with Ryan, my dogs, and an awakened Self who can still enjoy the beauty of this life.

The message I'd finally received was that I'm safe. I'm loved and whole. I'm a being made of love and light. I'm a child of God, of creation. I can create my own reality and my own future reality. I can manifest my deeper dreams into existence. My body's a way for my soul to express itself in higher vibrations of joy, love, and peace.

Your outer self-concept makes up everything you believe your body is capable or incapable of. Your body serves as a house for your soul to experience this life on earth. Some of that experience may be painful, but it doesn't add up to all that is you.

Your soul is space, expansion, and immensity, and the one thing it needs most is the freedom to expand, to reach out and embrace the infinite. Your soul has no restrictions or limitations. It resists being fenced in by rules and obligations. This part of you is part of something much bigger, beyond what you can see. You can reorder your life by choosing spirit over the illusion of physical circumstances.

You may reach a point of darkness where all hope feels lost. Surrender to it, and you will find the light, for it is in those darkest hours that you are most open to receiving it. In this space, love is greater than fear. Fear is a blockage to freedom. Turn to love. This encompasses compassion for yourself and for others.

I have a true semblance of life with less pain, of one with peace with endo. It's possible for you, too. You are a divine creation with the ability to heal. Do you believe it? Once you connect with that divine part of you, your soul existence, your life will change. I'm here to help show you how, and to support you along the way.

I hope to bring some light to your life. I'm shining it at you now, and I can feel it reflecting back. You were meant to read these words, as I am meant to share them. We're connected for a reason. I think you've been looking, too, for that spark of hope in the darkness. You want to know that it's possible to heal.

You need to look no further. What you need isn't "out there". The answers are within you. Stop looking for the light. Turn yours on. Take off your shades. You are beautiful. You are the light. Connect to it, and watch as miracles start to happen.

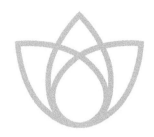

26. Connect

"When you dwell in an energy of positivity and power,
you become a magnet for miracles."

~ Gabrielle Bernstein, The Universe Has Your Back:
Transform Fear to Faith

When you live with pain, it's hard sometimes to explain that the experience to others. It's hard for others to understand. It's helpful to connect with ladies that do. Maybe that's why you're reading this book right now. You're seeking out further emotional connection. You want to feel heard and understood. We all do.

Endometriosis led me to using my voice, and speaking up. I've shared intimate details with you here because I know you can probably relate to some of it. I've lived it and been witness to it, and I can tell you after six years in the Peace with Endo community that there's power in holding space for others who need healing, especially when it's among other amazing, strong, compassionate women who are there to lift you up.

There's power in community of women, especially when it's collected under this pulling desire and intention for peace. All the work I'd done with Kate over the years showed that my roots were shaky. I needed more support. I was grateful that I've been able to find much of this within the endo community, but I wanted to take that a step further.

I craved having real conversations about the truth of living with endometriosis. These intimate conversations came up in my one-on-one coaching calls. One of the biggest benefits I saw with my clients was the space to release whatever they needed to. We don't always have space to talk about all that comes up with endo. It's easy for those emotions to build up inside.

When you're not free to speak your truth, the energy gets blocked up in your throat space. This leads to issues with your thyroid, tonsils, and sinuses. It's your voice. It's your source of communication, trust, and speaking your truth. I feel the pain in the endo community from not being heard. I recognize that this is a deep wound. Unfortunately, many times women's pain isn't taken seriously in the doctor's offices. It's brushed aside, or is quick to be silenced with pills and, dare I say, poison. These additives dull your senses and your pituitary gland. They numb your intuition. Please her me when I say: it's not the only way.

As a highly sensitive empath, I pick up on the emotions within the endo community. I continue to feel your pain and want to help you feel better, if you're open to receiving it.

When we rise together, our collective energy rises. Every "one" is connected. We're all flowing with life force. It's energy. It's everything. With it we impact each other.

This goes back to Carl Jung's teachings on the collective unconsciousness. Jung theorized that our personal psychology is part of a collective psyche, which moves according to laws entirely different from those of your own consciousness. Within our new awareness, we have a direct connection with a united field of energy.

Through prayer, meditation, positive intentions, and joy, we can change the collective unconsciousness and create a ripple effect of peace in the world, or at the very least within the endo community. This ripple effect has been proven with studies of the Maharishi Effect. Maharishi Mahesh Yogi was a spiritual teacher who founded the Transcendental Meditation movement. He predicted that if one percent of the population meditated, it would produce measurable improvement in the quality of life for everyone.

He believed that raising the vibration of this collective energy field with joy and calming energy would bring peace and harmony to the rest of the community. When people meditate together with shared intentions for peace, their alpha brains synchronize. This allows people who do not meditate to still receive the same properties in their subconscious.

You have the power to alter the energy field of this collective unconsciousness. With positive energy we can help bring healing to those around us. Once you tap into this power, others will feel elevated by your presence. It's time to step into your power. You can have a much bigger impact than you think.

All of this inspired me to create Peace with Endo Connect, an online membership community of endo sisters that provides face-to-face support sessions, group meditations, and continuing education for women who are interested in managing endometriosis with a natural, holistic approach of healing body, mind, and spirit. This space is safe, and allows you to express yourself, to say what's on your heart, to release any emotions that are weighing you down. It's space for you to let go.

This is space to find your tribe. To come together and raise the vibe, to lift the collective consciousness. To meditate together, learn from each other and provide support to hold you up when you feel like you're falling. This comes in alignment with the knowing that collective energy is powerful.

Do you want to join us in changing the ripple of energy and raise the vibe? If this resonates with you, I invite you to join us there. You can learn more at peacewithendo.com/connect.

By sharing my voice with you here, I bridge a connection with you. I hope it's one that continues.

Much Love.

27. Action Steps

Here are some clear action steps that you can take on your own journey of exploration into the energetics of endo.

1. De-clutter. Get rid of things you no longer need. Clear space. When you let go of things that don't bring you joy, you open up space for new energy.

2. Get clear on how you want to *feel*. Write out three to four feelings and put them in a spot where you'll see them every day. Use these as a guide as you set goals and intentions for yourself.

3. Be aware of the workings of your mind. Create space to observe your thoughts. Know that these thoughts are not you. Connect to the true "you" that's listening to these thoughts.

4. Make space for alone time. Even if it's only a few minutes a day, make space to re-connect to yourself. Do some focused breathing. Feel as you feel.

5. Discover your natural strengths. When you know what you're naturally good at, this helps you find purpose and direction with your life. I highly recommend taking the Gallup StrengthsFinder test. (When you buy the book *StrengthsFinder* you get access to the test).

6. Uncover your biggest underlying fear. To help with this, I highly recommend the writing exercises in the book, *It Didn't Start with You* by Mark Wolynn.

7. Release the tension in your pelvic space. There are different hands on therapies to help with this. Pelvic floor therapy is one, or you can do your own vaginal massage as outlined in Tami Lynn Kent's book, *Wild Feminine*.

8. Acknowledge the pain. Be present with it. Feel the feelings, all of them. When you put attention on the pain, the intensity actually lessens. It takes your mind out of the equation. To help with this, I have a free meditation for pain that you can download at peacewithendo.com/meditation-for-pain

9. Connect with Mother Nature. Feel the earth on your feet, or the sand between your toes. Experience the majestic view of the mountains, or time among the trees. Disconnect from your electronics and re-connect with your Self.

10. Shift to an energy of receiving. The best way to receive is through meditation. Take at least ten minutes to be still. Before starting my morning meditation, I set a verbal intention: *I am open to receive. I am open to receive love. I am open to receive guidance. I am open to receive love and abundance.* Remember that it's okay to receive help and to ask for it.

11. Balance your chakra energy. You may need to seek someone who can help you with this. I do offer this as a long-distance service if you want someone well versed in endo and infertility. I'd love to connect. Find out more at peacewithendo.com.

12. Consider hands on energy work like Reiki. This helped me so much, and I've seen many other endo sisters have success. Seek out recommendations in your area, or as it was for me, open up to receive and see who comes into your path.

13. What gives your life purpose? What helps you initiate forward thinking, beyond your existing circumstances? Take hold of something you feel positively about, imagine the outcome, and take action to make it happen!

14. Use your voice. Talk, sing, hum. All of these actions stimulate your throat chakra and your vagus nerve, which plays a big role with your nervous system and pain management. Let your voice be heard!

15. Get creative! When you create, you open up connection to your higher Self and allow energy that needs to move to leave you. Creativity is a way to bring your soul into your physical existence. If you don't know what to create, think back to your young eight-year-old self. What did she like to make back then?

16. Fascia release therapy can help release tension and pain in your body. Fascia serves as a bridge to the mind/body connection, so it can help release trapped emotions too. Different hands on therapies include deep myofascial massage, Maya massage, and Kinetix.

17. Stimulate the energy of joy. Do more of what makes you smile, laugh, and have fun! Life is short. Try not to take things too seriously, love.

28. Reading List

The following books helped me along the way:

The Life-Changing Magic of Tidying Up by Marie Kondo

The Desire Map by Danielle LaPorte

The Untethered Soul by Michael Singer

The Highly Sensitive Empath: Feeling Skinless in a Sandpaper World by Gigi Miner

StrengthsFinder by Tom Rath

It Didn't Start with You: How Inherited Family Trauma Shapes Who We Are by Mark Wolynn

Anatomy of the Spirit by Dr. Caroline Myss

Wild Feminine by Tami Lynn Kent

Women Who Run with the Wolves by Dr. Clarissa Pinkola Estes

The Universe Has Your Back by Gabby Bernstein

The Sophia Code by Kaia Rae

Angels in My Hair by Lorna Byrne

Medical Medium by Anthony William

Living in the Light by Shakti Gawain

Man's Search for Meaning by Viktor Frankl

Miracles Happen: The Transformational Healing of Past-Life Memories by Dr. Brian Weiss

Pocket Guide to Spirit Animals by Steven Farmer

Letting Go: The Pathway to Surrender by David R. Hawkins

White Hot Truth by Danielle LaPorte

The Moses Code by James F Twyman

Acknowledgements

There was a lot of energy that went into the writing and publication of this book. I extend much love and gratitude to the following...

My husband, Ryan, for being the biggest supporter of my writing and dreams. Thank you for always being there to listen to my thoughts, and inspiring me to express my truth.

My Mom and Dad for being there during this journey of writing, for sharing your stories with me, and for being examples of love and grace.

My soul sister, Kate Patchett, for all the healing, guidance and inspiration you bring to my life. My life has transformed because of you. I'm forever grateful.

Bethan Louise, Cindy Ellen, and Karla Kueber for bearing witness to vulnerable pieces of my healing journey. Further love to Bethan for reading one of the first drafts of this book! I appreciate your support and motivation along the writing journey.

Kristy Graham for introducing me to energy healing through Reiki and for being the one I can talk to about all that comes up along the healing journey. I value your friendship and presence in my life.

Steena Marie for introducing me to the divine feminine and for shifting my entire world! You are amazing and inspiring. I'm blessed to have come into your path.

My editor Leah Campbell who was the first to read what was a vulnerable first draft. Thank you for shaping it into something much better! I appreciate your honesty and perspective from a fellow endo sister and one who's been through the trenches of infertility.

Melissa Binkley who continues to inspire me with the work she does in the world with women who've experienced sexual trauma. Thank you for the kindness you've extended to me and for connecting me with Jo Schaublin, my amazing editor.

Jo Schaublin for smoothing out my words and inspiring me to believe that this book in your hands now is worthy of reading! I admit I had many doubts along the way about putting it out into the world. Jo, you came into my life at the perfect time. I'm grateful for you.

I extend love to my endo sisters who are on this quest to find #peacewithendo. I love being witness to your healing journey and to watch the transformation that can unfold, if you allow endo to serve as your greatest teacher. I know how lonely this disease can feel, and I would not be here today had it not been the connections I've made with my endo sisters online. I'm grateful for *you*.

Connect with Aubree

As a certified wellness coach, best-selling author of *From Pain to Peace with Endo* and leader of the #peacewithendo movement, Aubree is deeply passionate about wellness and inspiring other women to reconnect with a life filled with love and positive rhythms.

Aubree offers one-on-one coaching sessions and chakra balancing sessions. She also offers group coaching programs through Peace with Endo Connect, an online membership for empowered ladies with endometriosis who want to manage the pain in a holistic way, are ready to show up and hold space for each other and who *believe* that it's possible to get better.

Aubree's programs are aimed at transforming your life through small, manageable changes. She creates a positive, motivating environment to help you reach a place of less pain, more energy and peace with endo.

Aubree is also available for speaking engagements on nutrition, healthy lifestyle, stress management and overcoming suffering.

Meet Aubree and stay in the know about upcoming happenings at peacewithendo.com.

Other books by Aubree

From Pain to Peace with Endo:
Lessons Learned on the Road to Healing Endometriosis

Lightning Source UK Ltd.
Milton Keynes UK
UKHW011820200519

343003UK00001B/44/P